SOUTHERN ILLINOIS UNIVERSITY PRESS
Carbondale and Edwardsville

COMMUNICATING
WITH YOUR
DOCTOR

R_x for Good Medical Care

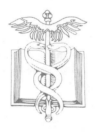

J Alfred Jones, M.D.

Gerald M. Phillips

Library of Congress Cataloging-in-Publication Data

Jones, J Alfred
  Communicating with your doctor.

  Bibliography: p.
  1. Physician and patient.   2. Interpresonal
communication.   3. Medical history taking.
4. Medical care.   I. Phillips. Gerald M.   II. Title.
[DNLM: 1. Communication—popular works.   2. Physician-
Patient Relations—popular works.   W 62 J77c]
R727.3.j65   1988   610.69′52   87-28379
ISBN 0-8093-1367-7

Contents

Preface

In this book, we do not evaluate medicine as a profession. Rather, we confront some of the major friction points between doctors and their patients and recommend practical steps patients can take to obtain quality medical care.

A great many medical schools are currently modifying their curricula to include effective communication skills and patient relations. We do not regard the process as a one-way street. To be most effective, the medical transaction requires that both doctors and patients are trained. By helping patients learn to get the most for each medical dollar, we can improve the medical transaction.

The advice in the book is derived from information we obtained from both doctors and patients. The questionnaires we used for this research may be found in the Appendix. The books to which we refer throughout the text are listed in the References. We studied middle-class patients who could afford medical care and the doctors most likely to provide it. Based on our study we will explain how you, the reader, can get the best care from your doctor.

Our thanks to the doctors and patients who provided us with information and to our colleagues who advised us and commented through the several drafts of the manuscript. We are grateful to our wives and families, whose patience throughout the project was most welcome. Special thanks to Professor Michael Hyde for getting the whole thing started.

COMMUNICATING
WITH YOUR
DOCTOR

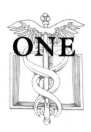

The Doctor-Patient Relationship

Great Expectations

When people are ill, they want action, reassurance, and care. They do not want delay and great expense. Everyone wants to feel good all the time, and most people believe that doctors are able to help when they do not feel well. Most people, in fact, 80 to 90 percent of those who visit doctors, are satisfied with the result. They are usually not annoyed until they get the bill. A satisfactory relationship between doctor and patient requires the exchange of useful information resulting in a good outcome. But, it is very difficult for patients to participate effectively, if they are naive, unskilled users of medical care.

To be a skilled user of medical advice, a patient must know something about the basics of human physiology, have a working medical vocabulary, be able to express symptoms accurately and clearly, and understand enough of what the doctor says to ask useful questions. Skilled users of medical services keep up to date on medical innovations and trends by reading, listening, and working conscientiously with their doctors. They must also have physicians who are also accurate and up-to-date, careful and considerate, good listeners, who are able to provide information accurately and intelligibly. Careful communication is a prerequisite for good medical care. At minimum this requires considerable contact between doctors and patients over an extended period of time. Years of association can lead to cooperation, understanding, and mutual confidence.

If patients could achieve this kind of relationship easily, this book would not be necessary. But, friction between doctors and patients often prevents the kind of understanding necessary for a satisfactory outcome.

Sources of Friction

The media. Medical practice fifty years ago is epitomized by the kindly old doctor in the Norman Rockwell print holding the patient's hand at bedside offering words of kindness and consolation. "Drink this, you'll be better in the morning." No one heard him mutter under his breath, "I hope." This image stands in contrast to the media image of the omniscient physician who is also heroic, handsome, administratively skilled, and capable of diagnosing and curing all ills. The clash between the images confuses users of medical services. False hopes and inappropriate expectations are a major source of friction between doctors and patients. Listen to the following:

CLIFFORD T. (PRESIDENT, MEDICAL EQUIPMENT
MANUFACTURING COMPANY), AGED THIRTY-SEVEN

We have just begun production on a multi-frequency laser device which, at some point should be effective in internal removal of intestinal polyps and tumors. It is a very hopeful technology, but it requires a great deal of testing before it can be used with humans. Furthermore, it is very expensive. No one can really afford to buy it. We are getting massive government support for the development and testing of the equipment, but when the newspapers got hold of the story they made it sound as though everyyone could come to their local clinic and get their cancers removed overnight without surgery. I want to tell you that the first prototype will not be tested with humans for three years. It will take us that long to get the first one going. I really wish the media would leave us alone because it is very hard to tell this story honestly to people who are dying and see in our work their last hope of survival.

When patients expect more than doctors can deliver, disappointment is guaranteed. Television dramas, for example, tell stories with precise beginnings and endings in exactly twenty-three or fifty-four minutes. But real ailments occur whenever and are diagnosed, treated, and cured within precise time segments. Most medical problems continue, get worse or better or disappear at their own pace, often independent of what both doctors and patients do. Doctors can help relieve the pain of acute illnesses as well as provide long term care for chronic illnesses. Their effectiveness demands considerable cooperation with patients.

Money problems. Another friction point is the image people have of doctors as being preoccupied with money. It is hard to be comfortable with physicians if you believe their motives are entirely monetary and devoid of humanitarian concern. Huge malpractice awards given by juries who perceive deep pockets in insurance companies, doctors, and hospitals rub salt in the wounds of doubt. Suspicion, whether justified or not, blocks the smooth and efficient exchange of information between doctors and patients. Some people are even afraid to seek medical help. They wonder, "Will I be the next victim of that money-grabbing so-and-so?"

MELINDA K., PH.D. (MEDICAL COMMUNICATION
SPECIALIST), AGED THIRTY-FIVE

Some people fear doctors so much they try to ignore them completely. That is, they concentrate on personal regimens and treatments. They run, they take vitamins, they refer to doctors as quacks, they complain that doctors are moneygrubbers who try to keep you sick. They are very irrational about it, but my studies indicate that at minimum, there are about one third of the people who need medical care and can afford it, yet still avoid it. Sometimes those people really pay a heavy price. When they get seriously sick they have no medical records and they do not know how to interact with their physicians. They have no one to manage their care.

Gossip. Finally, everyday gossip and social commerce litter the pathway to satisfying doctor-patient talk with hurdles difficult to clear. Stories from "he literally saved my mother's life" to "I thought he'd kill me" abound in every family, neighborhood, and social set, stirring pride or resentment in everyone within earshot.

Some stories must certainly be true, while others only the most enthusiastic gossip would embrace. But when people are afraid to use doctors, they may endanger themselves with self-doctoring. Books and magazine articles recommend diets of roots, nuts, berries, and seeds guaranteed to keep us healthy and sexy into our eighties; compulsive exercise, starvation diets, megavitamins, and major life modifications like "wellness" and "actualization" are offered as panaceas for all human miseries. Uninformed chitchat can seriously distort expectations people have about health and sickness.

Our friendly, local pharmaceutical supermarket has rows and rows of shelves filled with remedies for heartburn, stomachache, headache, arthritis, bursitis, constipation, diarrhea, impotence, infection, nagging backache, the jitters, the bots, the nines, the yellows, not to speak of the spavins and the yaws. An extraterrestrial visitor marooned in such a market could scarcely be faulted for believing that humans lead sick lives. People recommend remedies to each other, often erroneously.

Communication. Though most people with long-standing relationships express satisfaction with their doctor, many people complain that they cannot communicate well with medical personnel. Some experts now estimate that about 50 percent of patients actually follow their doctor's advice. The problem of defective communication between doctors and patients does not seem to be associated with age, intelligence, gender, economic status, race, or religion. Experience with the same doctor over time seemed to be the main influence for effective communication. Patients without a regular doctor often complain that doctors ask too many questions and take too little time to explain and give support.

Communication and the Doctor-Patient Relationship

Effective communication requires care and precision from everyone involved. The most frequent patient complaints are 1) their doctor patronizes them by using technical terms; 2) it takes too long to get an appointment; 3) they spend too much time in the waiting room; 4) the doctor does not explain what he is doing when he conducts an examination; 5) the doctor keeps them in suspense waiting for test results; 6) the doctor is unsympathetic to their human needs.

Doctors respond by asserting that they cannot provide the time and emotional commitment some patients seem to need. Doctors claim they are under pressure to care for great numbers of patients and they must remain detached in order to offer objective medical judgments. Doctors charge that their patients do not listen carefully and tend to waste available time with pointless chatter and trivial questions.

The problem seems to arise from the roles played by doctors and patients. Humans start life self-centered. As they mature, they learn to submerge their egocentrism in order to form social relationships like friendships and families. But this skill seems to disappear when people seek care from a physician.

The purpose of a doctor visit is self-centered. "Help me" is the message. The visit is sought by the patient for his or her own welfare. The doctor provides the service sought. Thus, the patient justifiably expects a full measure of commitment and concern. At the same time, however, the physician thinks good doctoring involves careful analysis and effective recommendations for treatment. The patient is emotionally involved with pain or discomfort and wants relief. The physician is involved with data and reasoning and often overlooks the patient's emotional concerns. Modulation of these human characteristics might eliminate some of the basic barriers to effective doctor-patient communication.

ALMA T. (DOCTOR'S WIFE, RETIRED
RECEPTIONIST), AGED SEVENTY-FOUR

We tried to keep the waiting room homey, you know. We had comfortable chairs and some good things to read. They came in once and tried to sell us piped in music but I couldn't see making the patients listen to that awful music. I had a tape deck and I played symphonies in the background. I knew everyone by name. Bill called them by their first name and they called him "Bill," or maybe "Dr. Bill." Back after the war, it was rough. Even an appendectomy could be touch and go. Bill tried hard to keep up with new inventions. He went to meetings and seminars and took courses and he was a good sur-

geon. *He really cared about those people. Even when he retired
he couldn't keep away from the office, and when he didn't do
surgery any more he did sore throats and warts or whatever the
folks brought in. They paid us as they could. Farm folks
brought us hams and things. But Bill used to say, "when I got
my science, I lost my priesthood." Bill was like a priest in the
early days. It was about all he could do. When he had better
tools and more knowledge, then it was all he could do to keep
up with the work. We gained a lot, but we lost a lot. I wish
there was some way to do it both ways.*

A Picture of Contemporary Medical Practice

Medical practice from the doctor's point of view:

STEVEN W., M.D., AGED FORTY-FIVE

*I really don't have much time for any one patient unless the
situation is serious. I am at the hospital before 7:00 A.M. every
day, seven days a week except for the few weekends I am off. I
am in my office at 9:30 A.M. every day and see patients til 4:30
P.M. with maybe a half hour for lunch when I can get it. Then
back to the hospital. I schedule twenty-five patients a day,
roughly allowing fifteen minutes for each, but there are always
five or ten people who must be seen or demand to be seen and
a few who aren't serious who are scheduled a day later. That
means I must shave time from patients who need less and give
it to patients who need it more. I don't think any of those patients understand the conditions under which I work, and I
don't have time to explain. I have to get done on time and get
back to the hospital for another hour or two before I get dinner. And then, all through the evening the phone rings.*

Medical practice from the patient's point of view:

SARAH B. (MOTHER, HOUSEWIFE, SECRETARY), AGED FORTY

*When I called for an appointment, the secretary listened to
my complaint and said I needed twenty minutes and that I
could come right away because there was a cancellation. I
drove down there like a maniac to be on time. Well, you can
guess that when I got there the secretary was now a reception-*

ist. *"The doctor was running thirty minutes late," she said. An hour later, I went into an exam room to take care of my cough.*

True, that poor man ahead of me was awfully sick-looking, clutching his chest and gagging, and he must have needed a lot of time, but the second lady that went in looked perfectly healthy. She shouldn't have taken sixty seconds. Why did I have to wait an hour? And then when I got in, the doctor asked me a few questions and checked my mouth and listened to my chest and hustled me right out with a prescription in my hand. "You'll be all right in a while," he told me. I got spun around so fast, I completely forgot my questions. I didn't know what the pill was or what it was supposed to do. I guess, since I didn't ask any questions the doctor thought I understood everything, but there was no time.

Lets take the interaction one step at a time to see where some of the problems arise. Here are the steps in virtually every doctor-patient interaction.

Patient	*Doctor*
1. I have a problem that requires medical advice.	1. I am trained to advise those who seek advice from me.
2. I choose a physician to whom I will bring my problem.	2. I am available for professional contact with patients.
3. I make an appointment to see the doctor.	3. I make an appointment to see the patient.
4. I appear for my appointment.	4. I see my patient.
5. I present my problem.	5. I listen to the patient, observe, check, test, examine records, and ask questions.
6. I provide information required.	6. I think through the problem and offer advice.
7. I listen to the advice, ask questions, and decide how to respond.	7. I record the information in the patient's records.
8. I pay the bill.	8. I process the payment.
9. I ask for help when I need it.	9. I respond to questions asked.
10. I report back results.	10. I wait to hear the outcome.

This sequence of steps represents a single problem-solving activity. There can be problems in any of the steps. 1) The patient may not understand his or her problem; the physician may not be qualified. 2) The patient may make an inappropriate choice of physicians. 3) The doctor may be overscheduled, the receptionist may interfere, the patient may not ask for an appointment properly. 4) There may be delay before getting in to see the doctor. 5) The patient may not phrase the problem accurately; the doctor may misunderstand; the examination may not be effectively performed. 6) The patient may ask the wrong questions; the doctor may provide wrong answers; the diagnosis may be erroneous. 7) The patient may misunderstand the advice, misuse the prescription, or not comply; the doctor may not record the information accurately. 8) There can be disagreement or embarrassment re: the payment. 9) The patient may not be able to reach the doctor with questions; the doctor may not respond to questions. 10) The patient may not provide follow-up information; the doctor may not use it adequately.

The medical collaboration depends not only on the skills of both parties but on two fundamental principles. First, the collaboration is voluntary. Although doctors frequently speak of "my patients" and patients of "my doctor," neither has a proprietary interest in the other. Patients are free, under most circumstances, to choose and change doctors anytime they like. Doctors, except under special circumstances, are free to accept or reject any person as a patient. Second, the relationship is morally based. Society sets standards of behavior for both parties. This morality is expressed in the statement "first, do no harm," taken from the Hippocratic oath. By definition, doctors are simply humans whose vocation is caring for other humans.

Learning to Be Doctored

MARVIN P., PH.D. (MEDICAL SOCIOLOGIST),
AGED THIRTY-FOUR

The late Irving Lee used to tell the story about the little boy who was being taken to the doctor by his mother for a shot. The little boy began crying as soon as he heard the news. His mother, a parental psychologist of no mean ability, told the lit-

tle boy, "now, darling, it won't hurt for a while. It won't hurt when you get there. It won't hurt while you are in the waiting room. It won't hurt until the doctor puts in the needle. Then it will only hurt for a minute, and then you may cry for a minute." The little boy seemed satisfied. He went to the doctor, and when he got his shot, he dutifully cried for a minute. On the way home he looked at his mother and said, "that doctor probably went to a bad school. He didn't hurt me at all." "Then why did you cry?" asked his mother. "Because you told me I was supposed to," the little boy said.

In the above example, the child's expectations are set by the parents before the visit. Whatever apprehension, confidence, pleasure, pain, or satisfaction the child feels about medical contacts will carry over into adulthood.

No one teaches children to choose a doctor, or the reasons for doing so. Going to the doctor is something that happens. In fact, most people grow up not knowing when they need to see a doctor. When they are sick, they are likely to scurry about asking friends for recommendations or choosing a name at random from the yellow pages. Often the decision is made on a basis of which doctor is close to home and available now.

AARON K., PH.D. (ANTHROPOLOGIST), AGED THIRTY-FOUR

People have special ways of relating to healers in every society. The medicine man always has special powers in the community. In America, doctors are accorded high status because we value the work they do and so we value them also. On the other hand, we often fear encounters with our doctors because they see us when we are at our weakest and they sometimes bring us bad news. Blood pressure, you know, is always highest in the doctor's office, a sign of the tension that exists in the typical patient who faces a medical contact.

The need to seek a physician becomes evident when the body becomes ill. A more rational decision about which physician to choose can be made, however, when the body is well. The process of choosing a physician is an act of consumership similar to selecting nutritious foods at the supermarket. It is not a simple act.

People learn a great deal about doctors by going to them and listening to others talk, but they are rarely taught how to select doctors or use them well.

The qualities a patient should seek in a good doctor are partly personal, partly professional. Courtesy and respect are components of all successful interpersonal relationships. In the medical relationship knowledge and skill are also important. An examination of the training doctors receive can provide some important insights into what a patient can expect.

Learning to Be a Doctor

The decision to become a doctor is sometimes made very early for those who are attracted by the adventure implicit in the practice of medicine. Parents and teachers often encourage children to think about being doctors. Medicine is a high-status profession that brings good income and a challenging professional life. Young doctors-to-be are usually upper middle class and high achievers in school. Recent efforts to draw ethnic minorities into medical schools have not made much difference, though the number of upper-middle-class women in medical schools has increased in recent years.

ANDREI K., PH.D. (MEDICAL SOCIOLOGIST),
AGED FIFTY-NINE

No matter how hard the medical schools try, they do not seem to be able to attract lower- or lower-middle-class people. Medical education is based on mainstream ideas like respect for school and social sophistication that seem second nature to those who live and learn in enriched environments. The few lower socioeconomics who get into medical school are often given special attention, for their skills are desperately needed by their people, but there are still not enough. Despite attempts by medical schools to attract them, not much has happened. And often those minority group members who do make it through medical school do not even want to return to their home communities.

To qualify for medical school, a student must have high grades from a quality school. Medical students are selected on criteria of academic accomplishment, social skills, and emotional stability. It is a highly competitive process, for medical schools have high standards and there are more good applicants than schools can possibly admit. Furthermore, most medical schools are committed to their students completing the program. They do not welcome potential washouts.

The prospective medical student must start qualifying for medical school from the first day of college. "A's" must be earned in the right courses. Science is emphasized, although most programs also encourage some work in the humanities and social sciences. To be taken seriously, a medical school applicant must do well on the Medical College Aptitude Test (MEDCAT) and be very near the top of his or her graduating class. Recent cutbacks in medical school admissions because of an oversupply of physicians have intensified the competition for places.

ANDREI K., PH.D. (MEDICAL SOCIOLOGIST),
AGED FIFTY-NINE

The selection process used by the medical schools guarantees that each generation of doctors brings in a new generation very much like itself. Students are continually pressured to comply with the rigorous procedures that characterize the practice of medicine. The ideal doctor displays attention to detail, detachment, analytical skills, coolness under pressure, and decisiveness. There is nothing wrong with this because the ability to make and test hypotheses is the hallmark of good clinical medicine.

Some medical schools try to enrich the curriculum with training in humanities and the arts. There is little resistance to this, because doctors have been exposed to the arts and literature in their homes and schools. Most are quite well rounded, actually. Many doctors have rich and active avocational lives and are not usually found on the golf course on their day off. It is important for patients to know that their doctors come from the best and the brightest and if anything goes wrong it is probably the result of things that happened after medical school.

First-year medical students learn they are entering a profession with special privileges and extraordinary responsibility. Their world is exclusively devoted to medicine. It engulfs students from the first moment until they begin practice. The implications of the commitment to work, seven days a week, all year, year after year, sink in only after training begins. This commitment distinguishes the medical student from all other graduate students. No other teaching/training system is so time-consuming for so long a time. It changes the student fundamentally and forever.

The medical school curriculum involves mastery of subject matter, learning responsibility to patients and accountability to superiors. Professors hammer knowledge of the scientific method, diagnostic techniques, and effective clinical treatment into students already softened to spongy readiness by four years of grinding in undergraduate school. The science of medicine is scooped up and fed in huge bites to the emerging doctor. The art of medicine is passed on by close observation of senior physicians; an apprenticeship in which students learn to imitate those who know.

Medical training is mostly conducted in the presence of patients. Students and residents assume responsibility early, but every history, physical exam, or clinical decision they make is carefully reviewed, criticized, corrected, and often redone by supervising physicians. Medical students must learn accuracy and responsibility. They must defend their decisions, and penalties for being wrong are often severe.

The curriculum is rigorous, both in subject matter and in clinical activity. It encompasses anatomy, physiology, pharmacology (how drugs work), diagnostics, and therapeutics. In addition, somewhere along the way, students gather a required pass into psychiatry, the closest thing to training in interpersonal relations that exists in medical training. Interpersonal relations with patients are learned through experience; mostly students model the behavior they see in their supervising physicians.

Real doctoring begins on the clinical rotations, six-week experiences on the wards and in the clinic. Real people with genuine disorders confront the student physician. The outcomes are not predetermined, often they are not positive. It is here the young physician learns to confront suffering and death.

Students must have the widest range of experience. That is why most medical training is conducted in large medical centers flooded with people with both common and unusual disorders. Many of these people cannot pay; few have regular doctors. They become teaching patients with whom young doctors can gain experience. If they could not become clinical subjects for medical training, many of these people would not be able to afford medical care.

The confrontation young physicians make with reality is often very hard. Note the following comments about medical training.

KEN W., M.D. (FAMILY PRACTICE), AGED TWENTY-NINE

Medical school was constant stomach trouble. I always felt tension about everything. I worried about doing and saying the right thing, to the patients, to the attending physician, to my friends, to my parents who were paying the bills. It seemed like everyone was on me all the time to find the right way to act. They never told you the right way, you had to find it and then you had to do it.

LOUISE T., M.D. (INTERNAL MEDICINE), AGED THIRTY-TWO

I lost all my social skills in medical school and residency. I didn't have a real date from my first year at ——— til I opened my office here in town. The real estate man who found my office for me asked me to have dinner with him. We went to a real restaurant and I found myself pushing open the door and sitting down before he could pull out the chair for me. I even took command of the ordering. By golly, I was a doctor. I had lost every other identity I ever had. I also did not have another date with him.

PHIL Y., M.D. (INTERNAL MEDICINE), AGED THIRTY

I am glad I came into this medical group because I don't think I know how to be alone any more. I got so used to watching the older doctors and learning what to do from what they did that I would just hate to be on my own. I need someone around to ask and it scares me that some day I will be an older doctor and some kid will be watching me and depending on me to figure out what to do.

Medical students must pass National Board Exams as well as their own school's subject matter exams. At most medical schools, students must pass part 1 of the National Board Exams to move from the second to the third year of medical school. To graduate, the student must pass National Board Exams, part 2. The prestige of a particular medical school often depends on what percentage of its students pass National Board Exams on the first try. Consequently, medical schools emphasize the subjects on which students are most likely to be examined. Pressure to succeed is intense. Failure to live up to the academic expectations of the medical school could mean career failure.

During postdoctoral residency, every effort is made to train students to avoid error. The dictum, "above all do no harm," is a constant superego and it is enforced by teaching and attending physicians who check every aspect of the resident physician's work.

Because the emotional strain is very great, most students learn to detach. In a teaching hospital, patients come and go. They are there because they need care and agree to participate as a teaching case. Poor people with serious diseases often get good medical care because they become cases that senior doctors can use to train resident physicians. The process of public review in which resident physicians are praised and blamed before their colleagues teaches them to concentrate on facts. The idea is to learn to do it right the first time! In fact, the pressure is so heavy that in mid-1987, many of the major big-city teaching hospitals began to revise their scheduling of medical residents in order to reduce long hours and emotional pressure in the interest of better patient care.

The word "internship" no longer applies to the first-year of postdoctoral training, since most students continue on for three to five years of training in some specialty. The length of postdoctoral training is determined by the requirements of the specialty the physician chooses. Even though most states allow an M.D. to practice after one year of postdoctoral training, hardly anyone does. Most authorities consider only one year of postdoctoral training insufficient. The knowledge and skill required by physicians demand at least three to five more years of training.

Resident physicians with some experience are given responsibility to teach younger physicians. For example, in internal medicine, i.e., adult diagnosis and treatment with medicines, the first-year resident physician will spend three months in the emergency room seeing acutely ill patients, three months on some specialty service (cardiology, endocrinology, nephrology, e.g.), and six months on the general medical wards where most adult diseases are found. During the second year, the internal medicine resident physician will spend another six months on the medical services, three months on specialty services, and three months in the medical outpatient clinics. The third year includes three months on ward services as a supervising physician, three months in medical clinics, and six months on services or specialties chosen by the resident.

What actually happens contradicts the media image of doctors closely attached to individual patients. Doctors in training dedicate themselves to learning the details of their profession. Patient loads are heavy and allow little time for personal contact. Resident physicians must be ready to answer questions from their supervisors about symptoms, test results, and responses to treatment. They must take responsibility for treatment recommendations. They learn to make emergency decisions and move rapidly. When has anyone seen a doctor who is not in a hurry?

Conditions really change very little when the doctor goes into private practice. The average doctor sees around 120 patients per week. Each must be given a fair share of time. In addition, doctors must make notes, keep records, make hospital rounds, attend meetings and continuing education classes, travel from home to office to hospital, eat lunch and dinner, and try to relax. Private practice does not materially alter the pressure.

Adjustment to a new professional life may be complicated by changes in personal life-style. Most doctors who have just completed their training face serious financial problems as they try to reduce the debts incurred paying for medical school. They have a real incentive to develop a steady patient flow and establish a solid financial footing. Sometimes to ensure regular income, young doctors will take on insurance physicals or service to social agencies and prisons to make ends meet.

Most young doctors come out of training $70,000 to $100,000 in debt. An office must be leased, furniture and examining equipment purchased, and personnel hired. Basic equipment might include examining tables, Holter monitor, EKG and lung function machines, laboratory equipment including microscope, sterilizer, cabinets and bottles, and the various lights, stethoscopes, sphygmanometer, syringes, etc. A conservative estimate for mostly used equipment is $50,000. New, it would cost $100,000. A receptionist-secretary and a nurse-assistant can cost roughly $40,000 including benefits and social security, more in competitive labor areas. Malpractice insurance is expensive. For an internist in a relatively middle-class community it can be as much as $4,000 to $8,000 a year. In larger cities, the price goes up. Obstetricians pay $60,000 a year in some communities. In addition, there are the customary business costs like taxes, rent, utilities, office supplies, and so on. Usually, doctors starting up will borrow enough money to live on and pay practice expenses for the first six months to a year. It is not surprising that many young doctors seem preoccupied with money.

There are some emotional adjustments to make also. In the community, patients no longer look like those in the teaching hospital. They are people the doctor grew up with. It is very difficult to detach from them. Few medical schools train doctors for the interpersonal relationships they will make in their regular practice. Some make excellent adjustments to the personal involvements of a regular patient load. Others compensate for their uneasiness through excessive detachment or authoritarianism.

The psychiatrist, Harry Stack Sullivan, believed that personality was made up of the set of interpersonal behaviors people learned to expect from others, and that people negotiated personalities to meet mutual needs. Doctors differ from each other, just like ordinary human beings.

The young doctor comes into practice with a personal and professional history. She must work out her "bedside manner" with each patient. No doctor can please everyone. Each patient must make careful choices in order to find a doctor whose professional skills he respects and whose personality he likes.

A Typical Practice

Except in emergency situations, doctors and patients interact in a professional setting: an office, clinic, or hospital facility. The contract starts with an appointment made, on the average, three days before the visit. The patient is with the doctor as long as the severity of the illness demands. When the examination is being performed, the doctor may be joined by some other professional like a nurse or technician. This is especially important when the doctor examines someone of the opposite sex.

The content of a medical visit varies little from person to person and time to time. The patient presents a problem, the doctor analyzes it and recommends a solution. The patient leaves with instructions and is told to call if "such and such" should happen. But the essential relationship lies in the crucial understanding between doctor and patient about what each is responsible for and how to judge a desirable outcome.

DR. N. (GENERAL PRACTICE), AGED FIFTY-FIVE

Did you ever notice when your toe hurts you keep bumping it. Most of the time you never even know you had a toe. Your feet keeping working, toes and heels and all and you do not think, "I have a toe and it is working." Sounds simple, doesn't it? But when you break that toe, look out, because your mind will be on it constantly. A friend of mine, a pathologist, pointed out that most of the corpses he examined had gall-stones. Not all of them complained about it when they were living. In fact, no one, not even the patient knew about the gallstones. It's like that with most medical conditions. When something gets annoying or painful enough so that people notice it, then a doctor gets called. Oh, sometimes people have strokes or heart attacks and they keel over and then someone has to treat them. But nobody knows they are sick until they complain that something is going wrong in their body. That's when they come to the doctor.

Barriers to an Effective Medical Relationship

Vocabulary. Simple misunderstandings about the meaning of words are a major barrier to effective doctoring. The most effective doctor-patient relationships are characterized by patients that understand some technical language and can ask productive questions.

GRETA K. (PSYCHOTHERAPIST) AGED FORTY-FOUR

I run a program for colostomy patients. It is a very interest-ing program. It started out to be a support group, you know, people who wear bags helping people who wear bags get ad-justed, a kind of Alcoholic's Anonymous thing. But what it turns out to be is training people how to talk about feces and urine, learning the terms for the holes in their body, learning to be comfortable with those words by using them in sentences that make sense to their doctors. It struck me that maybe some of those people had symptoms they couldn't talk about that might have delayed their visit to the doctor and maybe pre-vented a cure, if you know what I mean.

Point of view. Different world views complicate communication. A doctor's life consists of a string of interruptions punctuated by occasional emergencies. Many people have jobs that provide them with long periods of uninterrupted work time during the day. They never have to deal with a life-threatening emergency. They can schedule a social event or go to the theater with every reason to believe they will not be interrupted.

Doctors, on the other hand, are on call day and night. When they are not on call they must provide coverage for patient emer-gencies. Both their social life and family life are frequently inter-rupted. Furthermore, the consequences of any mistakes they might make can be very grave. Because they must see so many people under trying conditions, physicians tend to remain detached from their patients. Their patients may want a close personal relation-ship, but few doctors have the emotional energy or time to become deeply involved with their individual patients. They must spend their emotional reserves carefully to meet the needs of all.

Stereotypes. It is the rare person who does not stereotype situ-ations and the people in them. Patients tend not only to think stereotypically about their medical conditions but to have expec-tations about the way their doctors will behave. The following case exemplifies the frictions that can arise through stereotyping.

MARLENE T. (HOMEMAKER), AGED FIFTY-ONE

I went to the doctor with a complaint about alternating con-stipation and diarrhea. I was getting preoccupied with my digestive tract, worried. I read the magazines and they told me about all the diseases I could have. My doctor started with a sigmoidoscopy in the office. Then he sent me off for a barium enema. Then he sent me off for a colonoscopy. Then he told me he couldn't really find anything wrong, that I had "irritable bowel syndrome," and he gave me a pamphlet and a diet list and told me to stop worrying about things. I really didn't know whether he was dismissing me because I had incurable cancer or whether he thought I was nuts. It's hard to stop worrying about things when you have things like that to worry about. And why did I have to have all those tests? Why did I have to have all those tubes shoved into my body? And why, if I had irritable bowel syndrome, didn't he give me something to relax my stomach? I read in a magazine about some drug that relaxes the stomach, and I read in another article about how bran was a great treatment for irritable bowel syndrome. Didn't he know about these things?

Marlene's doctor studied her case with the best available scientific methods. He got a good idea of what was wrong from Marlene's history. He checked carefully to rule out serious disease, and he offered Marlene a clear diagnosis with reasonable certainty.

Marlene, however, failed to ask questions. She did not ask why the tests were performed, nor did she inquire about the results. When her situation was diagnosed, she did not ask for an explanation. She was so locked in to her worries that she failed to talk when she had the chance.

She did not examine the encounter until it was over and did not think of her questions until it was too late to ask.

Her doctor, no doubt, could anticipate that Marlene would have questions, but he could not know what they were. All he could do is provide basic information about her condition and how to treat it. When Marlene failed to call back, he assumed everything was all right. She could have asked about what she read in the magazine, or she could have examined the diet list she was given. If she had, she would have discovered it was a high-fiber regimen. In short, if Marlene had had a more realistic, nonstereotypical image of her doctor, she would have been a better-informed user of medical care.

Sharing information. The initial burden of providing information in the medical transaction falls on the patient. The patient's complaint guides the doctor in subsequent investigation. The process of providing information is often complicated by the fact that patients may be worried and emotional about their condition. The doctor must extract precise information to guide her examination by following standard procedures for history taking and diagnosis, and she must ask questions in patterns to link up elements of the patient's report. Adapting to the particular emotional state of the patient without subverting the accuracy of the examination procedure can prove difficult.

Patients are fairly consistent in the questions they have. They want to know what they have and how serious it is, how badly it will hurt, whether they will recover, and what the doctor is going to do about it. Patients often feel reluctant to ask questions for fear of looking naive or stupid. The doctor, on the other hand, may answer the patient's questions in medical terminology, without realizing the patient does not understand the language and, thus, will miss the significance of the doctor's answers.

It is even more difficult to persuade patients to comply with recommendations. Once the doctor has made a diagnosis and given recommendations for treatment, patients are responsible for their own care. But many patients do not understand what effect a treatment should have or how quickly it should work. They may expect to be cured much more rapidly than is possible and blame the doctor when they don't feel better soon enough. But once a patient leaves the office, the doctor has no way of knowing whether the patient followed the advice. Our studies show that patients ignore their doctor's advice 30 to 40 percent of the time.

Medical costs. The cost of medical care is a major barrier to productive relationships between doctor and patient. A great many people fail to seek the medical care they need because of their fear of the bill. Potential patients often overlook the fact that medical practitioners make their living by charging fees for services rendered. Doctors are often reluctant to admit that their patients may resent their profiting from illness. But, medical practice is a reciprocal relationship. The doctor does not dole out advice or administer treatment to a passive body. The patient must participate in both diagnosis and treatment. Sigmund Freud used to advise young doctors that the therapeutic alliance would not be successful unless the patient paid. Payment, Freud believed, would convince the patient of the value of the service and motivate cooperation. The fee-for-service model of doctor-patient relationships contains the potential for consistent complications.

CONSTANCE M. (HOUSEWIFE), AGED THIRTY-FOUR

My husband brings home a good salary, and I work one day on the weekend, and we have health insurance. Still, it is $200 deductible, and it only pays 80 percent of care outside of the hospital. So, if all of us get sick, that's $1,000 a year before we even start getting anything back. We just try not to get sick at all. There have been a lot of times I've wanted to call the doctor but didn't. With three kids, if I called the doctor for every little ache and pain, I'd be $1,000 out very quickly. That's our recreation money, and it's no fun going to the doctor.

Constance can probably afford more care than she seeks. She may not understand what her insurance policy provides, or she may assign low priority to medical care. Most people with insurance coverage can afford the medical care they need. Some people who can afford medical care do not seek it because they believe other expenditures are more important.

The financial issue cannot be avoided. In the United States most medical care is provided by private practitioners. The American people have traditionally defined the medical relationship as a confidential transaction between doctor and patient and have valued the personal contact. As a society we have taken extraordinary measures to fund medical care. Third-party payment, group practice, welfare programs, and community action have all been built on the premise that medical care is a private and personal transaction between doctor and patient. The cost of medical care should not deter those who need it from seeking it.

The stress of illness. Being sick is very unpleasant. It is an interruption in life and a physical and financial inconvenience. Even a short office visit may involve time off from work, travel across town, sitting in a crowded waiting room, sometimes for a brief and inconclusive visit. A chronic medical condition, surgery, or a long hospitalization can easily deplete your financial resources, change your life-style, and halt your career, to say nothing of pain and tension involved in the illness. A medical encounter may be routine to the physician; to the patient it may be a total catastrophe.

Michael Hyde, a specialist in medical communication, describes serious illnesses as "breaks." An acute condition disrupts life continuity. It is not natural for people to sit on a cold examining table with their clothes off while another person looks into their body apertures. It is not natural for people to lie on a hospital bed with tubes coming out of their arms and nose. People feel the indignity of having their bodies violated and their natural life flow interrupted. Patients worry about money, loss of work, permanent disability, loss of important body functions, how their loved ones will respond, what is going on at home, and what the future holds. If the illness becomes chronic, it may require permanent life changes.

For the doctor, critical and life-threatening problems are routine. Each case requires careful scientific analysis in a limited amount of time. No one patient can be permitted to interfere with the time and consideration given to another. The doctor is always involved in weighing the gravity of one case against another. This process of triage sometimes requires her to make agonizing decisions about how to divide up her expert time.

Patients can easily misinterpret this detachment. They do not really know what other cases their doctor is balancing at any given moment. Her preoccupation with a life-or-death situation somewhere else may make it seem she is uninterested in the case at hand. This difference in perspective can seriously strain the relationship between doctor and patient.

ALAN McT., M.D. (CHRONIC DISEASE SPECIALIST),
AGED FORTY-TWO

I treat people with long-standing diseases. When I was in regular practice I noticed that there is a change when a patient discovers he has a chronic disease. Most patients are occasional. They come in for this and that and there is no continuity. But once you have a disease that requires regular attention, you have to establish a new relationship with your doctor. Now that I see only chronic patients I discover I have to know a lot more about them as individual human beings. When you are treating a cold you are treating a cold but when you treat arthritis you are treating a person. Sometimes doctors and patients alike are not aware of this change. I urge patients to be aware of their own changing needs and take steps to get their doctor to adapt to them.

Intimacy. Few human relationships involve sharing intimate secrets like the doctor-patient relationship. Ordinarily, sharing of intimacy makes both people vulnerable. But this is not a relationship of ordinary sharing. Doctors rarely disclose intimate details of their lives to patients. Patients tell their doctors a great deal about their personal lives, which their doctor is obliged to keep confidential. A major barrier to effective doctoring is patient reluctance to disclose important details of their physical and emotional lives. Doctors must train their patients to become participating partners in medical treatment by teaching them how to communicate important information.

Goals for the medical encounter. In an ideal system, this is what patients seek in return for their medical dollar.

—The doctor would monitor their bodies, keep records of how their systems work, and recommend suitable treatments.
—The doctor would keep up to date on the latest innovations and trends to take advantage of the widest range of possible treatments.
—The doctor would stay in contact with patients who have chronic conditions to ensure maximum comfort.
—The doctor would represent patients when contact with specialists is necessary, supervise any hospitalization, and co-ordinate all medical treatment.
—The doctor would show concern for patients as human beings and give them necessary time and information.
—The doctor would be available when needed and provide qualified substitutes when absent.
—Patients would also be obligated to help their doctor meet their goals.

—Patients would be alert to their physical conditions and be able to give accurate information when needed.

—Patients would be considerate of the pressures placed on their doctors and learn when it is appropriate to request medical services.

—Patients would accept their responsibility to pay for services rendered.

Doctors report that they like "cooperative" patients. A cooperative patient gives accurate information, doesn't waste time, listens carefully and asks good questions. *The best doctor-patient relationship is one in which a maximum of information is exchanged in a reasonable time.*

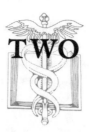

TWO

Understanding the
Medical Profession

What Do Doctors Do?

The partnership you and your doctor form is most effective when your physician is competent and you are cooperative. But there is another important quality of a good medical relationship called "bedside manner." This phrase refers to the nature of the personal relationship a doctor develops with each of his patients. An intelligent user of medical care has reasonable expectations about what doctors are able to do, understands how they do their work and what you as a patient can reasonably expect from them in the way of "bedside manner."

We strongly recommend that you have a personal physician with whom you can build a relationship. It is potentially dangerous to go from doctor to doctor without having someone coordinate and interpret information for you. Your goal should be to find a competent doctor with whom you are compatible. Understanding how medicine is practiced in the United States provides a basis for identifying such a doctor.

The contemporary practice of medicine. In virtually every "Star Trek" episode, Dr. McCoy, jocularly referred to as "Bones," passed a "scanner" over sick creatures, humanoid and otherwise, read a diagnosis dial, and prescribed just the right treatment for an immediate cure. Because he does his job so rapidly, Bones has time to have rollicking adventures with Captain Kirk. Today's doctors and patients want Bones' perfect diagnosis and rapid cure, but they are far from having it. Their equipment is only ordinary, hard and time-consuming to use, with much less to offer in the way of cures.

Medicine today is partly art, partly science. A half century ago, the best doctors had to offer was bedside manner. Diagnosis was uncertain and treatment was largely made up of traditional folk remedies. Vaccines, sulfa drugs, antibiotics, insulin, organ transplants, X rays, sophisticated laboratory analysis techniques, and computerized diagnostic equipment, among other things, have, over the last fifty years, revolutionized the practice of medicine.

Today's doctor is an applied scientist. He synthesizes generalizations about human physiology with his personal knowledge about individual patients. Humans are often harder to understand than the diseases that afflict them. Medical problems often have mysterious ways of revealing themselves, unique to individual cases. Doctors must make connections between what they see and what they know.

We take a great deal for granted about medicine because we have learned from the experience of others. Consider, for example, that diabetes was first diagnosed by Egyptian physicians who noticed that sweet tasting urine was associated with a variety of symptoms. No one accepted the germ theory of disease until midway through the nineteenth century. The enlightened scientists of France responded to Louis Pasteur with derision and ostracized him when he told them invisible organisms could cause serious disease. The idea that yeast could kill those germs was equally bewildering.

Your doctor must understand you as a person as thoroughly as he understands physiology in general. Most doctors are trained to listen carefully, take good notes, and make diagnoses with reasonable accuracy. Most find it somewhat more difficult to explain to patients what they have done, how they did it, and what it means. The following case illustrates how doctors make connections.

QUENTEN J., M.D. (INTERNAL MEDICINE), AGED FIFTY-FOUR

Here is a typical scenario. A patient tells me he has a "pain in the ear." I ask him to describe the pain and he tells me it is "sharp." I ask him some more questions and discover it is recurrent and associated with coughing and sneezing. I look in the ear, nose and throat and see that they are red. The irritations look like a general infection. I see bulges in the eardrum that indicate a rather severe ear infection. I do a test in my office for evidence of streptococcus infection. The test is inexpensive and if it is positive I can treat the problem with antibiotics. The test is negative, so I have a choice. I can take a culture and try to find out what is bothering the patient. I can prescribe a broad spectrum antibiotic, or I can tell the patient to go home, "there's a lot of this going around." I have seen a lot of it lately. I choose the medication, give the patient some advice that might help his symptoms, send the culture off, and wait for the results. By tomorrow, there may be something more I can tell my patient.

Forming a clinical hypothesis and testing it, a process referred to as the medical model, starts with the doctor's listening to you and observing your physical signs. From this, he generates an initial hypothesis about you, based on what he knows in general. He takes information from your history, the examination, the records, medical tests, and any other useful source so that, eventually, he is able to define your problem, propose a likely cause, and recommend some action.

Reasonable expectations. Understanding how your doctor does her work will enable you to set reasonable expectations for the encounter.

DR. MADELINE C. (GENERAL PRACTICE), AGED FORTY-FOUR

My patient Otto V. is a worker at one of our local factories. He came to me with complaints about stomach pain. I took his history and ordered several tests and made a clear diagnosis of a duodenal ulcer. I prescribed Tagamet and told him he could stay with his regular diet. I urged him to give up smoking and cut down on drinking and to get a bit more rest. I was very careful in explaining this program to him. I gave him a booklet on ulcers and what caused them so he could understand his condition. Mr. V. seemed quite bright. He asked questions about his problem, repeated my instructions back to me accurately and I had every reason to believe that he understood. But he has phoned me three times and come back twice because the treatment is not working. I do not want to put him through the tests or have gastroscopy (test to look into stomach) again so soon, but I believe he is not following my recommendations even though he seems to understand exactly what to do.

OTTO V. (MACHINIST), AGED THIRTY-NINE

I did everything Dr. Madeline C. told me to do. I have taken those pills according to instructions. I stopped smoking at once and I drink no more than two beers a day. I am even eating better. I took my wife's Weight Watchers manuals and I am sticking to their diet because it seemed to me it was healthier than the diet I was eating. But I still get the pains. I simply do not believe these pills are doing me any good. I wonder whether Dr. Madeline C. knows what she is doing.

Both Dr. C. and her patient could be right. Mr. V. may think he is following instructions, but Dr. C. cannot evaluate it because she does not know exactly what he is doing. It is possible that tensions in his life affect his condition. He may actually be improving objectively, but to confirm this would require some uncomfortable and expensive tests. Furthermore, Mr. C. may have forgotten to report that he is taking six aspirin tablets a day for his headaches, which perpetuates the problem.

On the other hand, Dr. C. may be expecting too much from her prescription. Her experience with Mr. V. as a patient may be too limited to know how he lives his life, or even that he doesn't consider aspirin a drug worthy of reporting. She only knows what he tells her.

Even the most conscientious doctors and cooperative patients have misunderstandings. For example, "Doctor, do I take two pills four times a day or four pills two times a day?" Anyone can misread or misinterpret instructions. When your doctor recommends you change your life-style, it is even more difficult. Your daily life can be ruined by attempting to diet or give up smoking when you don't want to. Your doctor can advise and persuade, but there is no way she can enforce these recommendations. Furthermore, she can never know how well a treatment is working, unless you provide that information.

History taking. History taking frames the doctor's work situation. The process starts with the assumption that the patient has a reason for seeking the doctor. The doctor must understand that reason, interpret it in medical terms, investigate it, and offer advice to solve the problem.

Unlike the fictional Dr. McCoy, real doctors do not have magic diagnostic gadgets. They must listen to what you say, see how you look, ask questions, and examine you. They need more than a list of your symptoms; they need to know in your own words what you think is happening to you. They cannot see into your world without your help.

KELLY J. (CHEF), AGED FORTY-FOUR

Most of the people I know have had this experience. I mean, you have a cough, you wake up with a cough and you don't want to cough germs into the food so you call the doctor. Some woman answers the phone and she says, "what's the matter" and you say "I have a cough" and she says, "well, we'll see when Dr. Squiffy has some time. Ahhh. How about Thursday." But it's Monday and you have to go to work. "Come on," you say, "I got the cough now. Maybe by Thursday it'll be gone, or I'll be dead." So she says, "Is it an emergency?" Now there's a question. How am I supposed to know if it is an emergency? I don't know anything about medicine. A friend of mine was stung by a bee once and somebody wanted to take him to the doctor and he said it wasn't an emergency and then he stopped breathing and he almost died and the people in the emergency room at the hospital bawled us out for not getting him there sooner.

Most doctors begin their examinations with questions about your condition, followed by a limited symptom-specific physical examination and tests. You are expected to provide accurate and complete information and ask pertinent questions. Your doctor should listen carefully and make connections between what you say, what he sees, and what he knows about the human body.

Usually doctors get a mundane initial report from their patients: "My throat hurts," or "I have been throwing up." But, doctors cannot stop at the obvious. The initial report must be carefully investigated. If your doctor knows you well, information from previous visits provides a clue to what is happening. Each patient has a unique pattern of symptoms. Some may get headaches during stressful situations at work. Others may get them before taking long trips. For some, a headache may be a very unusual occurrence.

If your doctor knows you well, he will perceive subtle changes in your body. He will interpret current events in the context of evidence from the past. "Is there anything unusual about the pain this time?" "Is it more severe?" "Do you feel anything else with it?"

Dr. Abner Y. (internal medicine), aged forty-eight

In most cases, patients have every reason to trust our experience, past and present. We know the range of disease and what their symptoms are, and we know what is happening with other people in the community. The phrase, "it's going around" is not silly. It happens all the time that a great many people come down with a disorder that produces similar symptoms at the same time. The best hypothesis is that they have the same thing. If we are talking viruses or bacteria, we know diseases are contagious. If we are talking people who work together or live together, we know the odds of contagion are high. I think doctors have to be careful, but I don't think they need to brood about an obvious diagnosis. It makes sense to try what is most likely to work first and then, if it doesn't work, explore other options.

When you come with a new complaint, your doctor requires new information. He will usually base his questions on the first thing you say. That is why it is very important for you to be be able to provide accurate, complete information about what you are feeling, when you feel it, and how bad it is. You must be able to answer your doctor's questions. He asks them for a purpose.

It is up to you to set priorities. In chapter 5 we provide you with an analysis form to use to prepare for a visit to the doctor. It will help you figure out what it is most important to say.

You may have trouble finding words to express your problem precisely, and your doctor may find it equally difficult to translate his ideas into words familiar to you. Shared experience, however, will help you create a common vocabulary. Following are examples of how this exchange is carried on.

ELIZABETH Y. (SECRETARY), AGED TWENTY-EIGHT
KEVIN V., M.D. (INTERNAL MEDICINE) AGED THIRTY-FOUR

MS. Y.: *When my period comes I bloat up; feel heavy and get the—ah—the runs, diarrhea, you know. Sometimes I bleed from down there, uhh, not where you make love—uhh, the other place, you know.*

DR. V.: *Did you look around the rectum to see where the blood came from?*

MS. Y.: *Ohh, no. I would never look down there, you know, by my privates.*

DR. V.: *What do you mean by "heavy feeling?"*

MS. Y.: *Well, I get this pressure, down below, like my thing's going to fall out. That's when all the fart—uhh, fanny burping begins. Doctor, is this normal or is this weird or something?*

ADELE V., PH.D. (COLLEGE PROFESSOR), AGED THIRTY-NINE

When I was carrying my second child, the senior obstetrician at the medical center was taking care of me. He was cautious, advised me against travel, continually admonished me to get a lot of rest, and watch my diet. He sounded to me like a man trying to avoid a malpractice suit. Obstetricians are particularly vulnerable, I hear. Then one day I went in and he was off and the senior resident in OB checked me over and said, "you have to be careful, your baby is in a compromising position." I always thought a "compromising position" was what you were in when someone walked in and caught you in the act and I giggled a little, and he got very serious and said, "look, your baby's life is at stake and so is yours." That was news to me. My regular doctor never told me. And the awful way to put it, "compromising position" indeed!

Some doctors find it difficult to talk about body processes. A few are embarrassed at the sight of the human body. Questions like, "Are your bowel movements normal?" are hard to answer, particularly since there is no definition of normal bowel movements. A better question would be, "Have you noticed any change in your bowel habits?" You can respond to a question like that simply by telling the doctor what has happened over the last few days. Competent doctors ask questions in a logical sequence. You may not, for example, see the connection between a potential heart condition and swelling in your ankles. It is important to ask about what you do not understand. Your questions can help the doctor in his examination.

What is bothering you? Where is it located? Is there anything that seems to bring it on? Can you describe it? Many adjectives can be used to describe pain, and doctors and patients rarely have a common reference point. You may assume that if something hurts you it would hurt someone else. But it is impossible for anyone else to experience your pain. Some people live their entire lives with serious medical problems and never complain, while others may report severe pain from physical conditions that appear trivial. There is no way to measure your pain objectively. Adjectives like "sharp," "dull," "throbbing," "piercing" are as objective as it is possible to get. A very effective way for your doctor to get information about your pain is to consider change: Is your condition worse, better, or unchanged?

To attain precision in diagnosis, your doctor may have to help you learn a more technical language. Each word must mean the same thing to both of you. To the physician, the word, "diarrhea," for example, means "watery stools more than four times per day. But if you normally have one bowel movement every other day, diarrhea may be three movements a day. Discussing everyday words can clarify a diagnosis in a way that X rays and blood tests cannot.

What else is bothering you? Complaints usually occur in groups. Every feeling is associated with other feelings. You may feel an earache, but a sore throat may be the source. You may have come to the doctor about your heart palpitations, but the crucial information may be that you are having difficulty breathing while trying to take a nap. Your recent quarrels with your boss or spouse may also provide a clue. Dr. W.'s story illustrates some of the problems that may come from an inadequate history.

DR. ANGELA W. (INTERNAL MEDICINE), AGED THIRTY-EIGHT

I learned the importance of an orderly history when I encountered Mr. C. Mr. C. was embarrassed about coming to a female doctor, but I guess I was the only one who was willing to give him an appointment in a hurry. He was having problems urinating, and I simply could not get him to tell me precisely what was wrong. He misinterpreted my questions. He looked away most of the time. From what he said I could have diagnosed a bladder or prostate infection or a kidney stone. I really didn't have enough information. I kept asking him questions and he would not respond to them. I asked him if it took a long time for his stream to get started. He seemed not to understand what I meant. He kept telling me "it kind of hurts when I, you know, wet." Imagine a man of fifty talking like that. I couldn't make a diagnosis based on that history and I asked him to drop his pants so I could at least check his prostate. He refused. I told him I couldn't make a diagnosis unless he let me examine him and he told me I was a lousy doctor. He left without paying the bill. Three days later, I ran into him again when I was making hospital rounds. He had been admitted as an emergency patient because of blood in his urine from passing a kidney stone. He didn't even tell the emergency room people he had been to see me. He told them he had never seen a doctor about it.

What is your past history? Your doctor needs a complete record of your ailments and physical development. Childhood diseases can help explain current difficulties. Your doctor should know about other physicians you are seeing and medications you are currently taking so that she can prevent dangerous drug interactions and overtreatment.

The way you have been treated by medical professionals in the past shapes your attitude toward your doctor. If your former doctors have intimidated you, you are likely to fear doctor contacts now. If discussing your sex life or bowel habits has embarrassed you in the past, discussing it now can be equally difficult. You may not want to reveal that you have been going to another doctor for fear your present doctor will feel threatened. But concealing this kind of information can cause genuine complications in diagnosis and treatment. In short, your doctor has no way of knowing what is on your mind. He can only respond to what you say.

Since time usually prohibits getting a complete history at the first visit, important details get filled in over time. Chapter 5 contains a form that you can use to gather information about your complete medical history.

Some important definitions. People can be sick in different ways. It is considered an emergency, for example, when patients' breathing becomes difficult, body temperature rises precipitously, they fall unconscious, bleeding continues despite all effort to stop it, or pain becomes unbearable. If this happens very quickly, it is called "acute."

Some acute conditions are not threatening. A sore throat that proves to be a strep throat happens suddenly but it rarely threatens your life. This affliction could be acute, but not an emergency. Also, treated or not, the strep throat eventually gets better by itself; it does not go on and on.

A disease that continues is called "chronic." A long-standing condition like diabetes or arthritis develops slowly, although the diagnosis may mean sudden changes in your life. Chronic ailments usually require regular treatment. Acute conditions occasionally herald a chronic problem. Any chronic condition can be punctuated with acute episodes.

The Physical Examination

What is done during a physical examination varies from patient to patient and time to time. Checking blood pressure, for example, is a brief, one-item physical. A thorough physical exam, "the physical," requires complex procedures and sometimes laboratory tests. Your doctor begins your examination the moment you arrive. How you look, walk, talk, smell; how you are dressed, sweat, or fidget usually provide more information than the rest of the short exam. Touching is also important. Feeling skin temperature, body shape, and organ placement gives more information. Finally, listening to the body with ear and stethoscope completes a thorough physical.

During a physical examination your doctor looks for some kind of impairment or variation from normal. Some impairments foreshadow serious events in the physical system that might endanger you; others are merely unnerving and pose no particular danger. The concept of "normal," however, can be confusing. Sometimes it refers to whatever is the case with most people. To a statistician, one-third of the cases slightly above the average and one-third slightly below are defined as normal; those outside the limits are abnormal. But abnormal is not synonymous with bad. Body temperature, for example is classified as "normal" when it is 98.6 degrees. On the other hand, there are some people whose usual body temperature is 97.2 degrees. For them, 98.6 might be considered elevated. The question your physician must answer is, does any observed abnormality indicate disease?

Dr. Theodore A. (opthalmologist), aged thirty-seven

Consider the simple evaluation we do when we prescribe glasses. It looks scientific doesn't it? We have all this complicated equipment we use to manipulate lenses in a very refined way. But in the final analysis, the burden is always on our patient to say which combination is better than which other combination. We keep looking and asking until we figure out which combination the patient prefers. This is probably the easiest example of physical examination. When a doctor is listening to a patient's chest with a stethoscope, he hears a great deal. He must decide whether what he hears is unusual, and if it is unusual, is it abnormal, and if it is abnormal, is it pathological, and if it is pathological, precisely what is it? That is a heavy burden to place on a human being using a simple piece of equipment. I have a real advantage over the other practitioners because I can at least ask my patients to pick one lens over the other. In most other examinations, the doctor makes all the decisions.

One final notion. I have always respected veterinarians, because they have to work with no talk at all. The cow cannot tell them where it hurts. Everything must be done by examination, visual examination, and the use of simple equipment. The point I am trying to make is how hard it is for the doctor to coordinate the history and the physical examination.

Description always precedes evaluation. Your doctor keeps records of your height and weight and notes changes in your appearance. Your vital signs—temperature, blood pressure, respiration, and heartbeat—are checked and recorded at each visit. Your doctor then classifies his observations into categories. If the inner lining of your nose is red, he must decide whether it is typical redness for noses in general, excessively red for you, and whether, in any case, it is red enough to be called an inflammation. He must then ascertain where the redness comes from and how far it goes. Redness in the nose can indicate a problem in the ear or throat. Your doctor decides whether the redness he sees is a sign of illness.

The importance of looking and listening. Medical training teaches doctors to look and listen carefully, taking nothing for granted. They seek details related to your symptoms, then search for possible causes. Simple observation as you enter the office begins the examination. The doctor looks for changes in your behavior and ask questions about what he sees. She will check on both your emotional and physical state to see if it differs from what she knows to be normal for you. Your handshake, for example, provides her with a sense of your musculature; the texture of your skin signals your general state of health. Looking into your eyes or touching your shoulder as she guides you to a seat provides information that can be used as a basis for questions.

A symptom is not a disease. It can be anything you consider a problem whether it differs from normal or not. Symptoms include feelings, thoughts, sounds, sights, smells, or worries. The following list describes what your doctor looks for during a physical examination.

1. Your doctor looks at you all at once to notice your way of standing, walking, breathing, talking, and how you hold your body. He looks for signs of bone, muscle, and joint disorders. He also gets a sense of your general state of health.

2. Your doctor looks in your ears, nose, and mouth because many diseases present findings in these areas, particularly in the back of the eye (retina) and the back of the throat.
3. Your doctor may feel your whole head to get a sense of your skull shape.
4. Your doctor feels the side of your neck to inspect lymph nodes (glands) that can indicate infection, to check your carotid arteries (the ones that supply blood to your brain) and neck veins for distortion.
5. Your doctor looks at and feels your spine for curvature and areas of tenderness.
6. Your doctor looks at the shape of your chest wall to see if you are breathing normally.
7. Your doctor listens to your lungs to identify normal breathing or sounds of fluid in the chest that can indicate lung disease or heart trouble.
8. Your doctor listens to your heart and feels the chest wall to detect abnormalities in heart function.
9. Your doctor examines breast tissue looking for lumps in men as well as women.
10. Your doctor examines your abdomen for irregularities, scars, tenderness, organ enlargement, and normal sounds of the bowel.
11. Your doctor examines your genitals for lumps, infection, enlargement, or discharge.
12. Your doctor examines your rectum for hemorrhoids, bleeding, irritation or pain. In men he feels the prostate for signs of enlargement or infection.
13. Your doctor looks at your extremities for signs of arthritis, deformities, limited motion, varicose veins, swelling, or artery disease.
14. Your doctor checks your reflexes and muscle motion to determine if your nerves are working properly.

If the combined history and examination do not provide enough information testing is necessary.

Specialists. Specialists usually have the equipment to perform some sophisticated tests in their offices, and many procedures can be performed on an outpatient basis in a local hospital. Complicated heart measurements like stress electrocardiograms, examinations of the digestive tract, X rays, scans, and MRIs require equipment that the typical doctor does not have in his office.

Some medical conditions are so complicated they require the services of a specialist. Specialists can be regarded as high-tech consultants to your personal physician. They provide assistance both in diagnosis and in treatment. Their focused knowledge and experience provide them with diagnosis-specific information that can be integrated into the other information about your condition. Many specialists restrict their practices to patients with particular types of diseases. They collaborate with general physicians who provide the rest of the required medical care. Some specialists, however, choose to include treatment of chronic conditions and may serve their patients as general doctors. Your personal physician can help you learn how to use a specialist. He should interpret information from the specialist for you in the context of your medical history and general physical condition. Currently, medical specialists are available in allergy, anesthesiology, cardiology, clinical medicine, dermatology, emergency medicine, endocrinology, epidemiology, family medicine, gastroenterology, gynecology, hematology, immunology, infectious diseases, internal medicine, nephrology, neurology, nuclear medicine, obstetrics, oncology, ophthalmology, otorhinolaryngology, pathology, pediatrics, physical medicine, psychiatry, pulmonary disease, radiation oncology, radiology, renal disease, surgery of various sorts, urology, and trauma medicine.

Laboratory tests. Vital signs require little time and equipment and can be checked in the office. Some doctors can also check your blood glucose level (to monitor diabetes), the condition of your anus (sigmoidoscope), or even do an electrocardiogram. Tests can be performed in a specialized laboratory on any body fluid or tissue. Blood, urine, feces, mucous, saliva, tears, and sweat can all be chemically analyzed. Your doctor coordinates the findings of these tests with the other information she has to clarify your medical problems.

Doctors select tests carefully to identify complicated conditions that resist other kinds of diagnosis. Laboratory tests, by themselves, rarely indicate a specific diagnosis, however. They are small pieces of the diagnostic puzzle. A biopsy, for example, might identify a tissue as pathological, but it cannot give any information about the distribution of the tissue or its impact on particular parts of the body.

The testing process can be irritating and it is always expensive. It cannot be hurried. Though your doctor sends for tests immediately, the results will probably not come for two days to a week, longer for more complicated tests that require specialized service. Furthermore, the costs of a complicated diagnosis can be prohibitive, particularly if you are not covered by medical insurance. Recently doctors have been charged with practicing "defensive medicine," that is, relying on extensive tests to protect themselves against malpractice charges. While there may be some abuses, in most cases, laboratory tests are well worth their costs.

Laboratory studies are sometimes used to establish base-line values for later comparison. Electrocardiograms (ECGs) and chest X rays in adults are often done when patients are well to make comparisons possible later on. Following are some of the more frequent laboratory tests and their purposes.

Urine analysis (UA): To test the state of the kidney and bladder as well as testing for diseases that produce substances in the urine.

Complete blood count (CBC): To count the various cells in the blood stream.

Lipids (cholesterol, triglycerides, HDL): These blood fats vary in many diseases and can indicate risk for hardening of the arteries.

VDRL: A syphilis test, commonly required for a marriage license.

Thyroid studies (T3, T4, T7, TSH): Blood tests to determine the state of the thyroid gland.

Cultures: Growing bacteria, viruses, or parasites from samples of body tissue or fluid to determine if infection is present, e.g., a throat culture for streptococcal bacteria (strep throat).

Liver tests (SGOT, alkaline phosphatase, bilirubin): To assess the health of the liver.

Kidney tests (BUN, creatinine): To assess the health of the kidneys.

Minerals (potassium, sodium, calcium, magnesium): Minerals in small quantities that are vital to body function can be lost in response to some medication, especially diuretics (water pills).

Medicine levels: Many good medicines are potentially toxic at levels close to those used to correct a problem. Their blood level is measured to make sure the dose is not too high or too low.

Blood sugar (serum glucose): An important measurement in the control of diabetes and related diseases.

In addition to these laboratory tests, X rays, body scans, and Magnetic Resonance Imaging are available to study the internal state of the body. X rays cost little compared to other procedures but are sometimes risky because of radiation. The more complicated procedures are quite expensive and usually done only when doctors suspect something very serious is wrong.

Diagnosis and Treatment

The most important part of the medical visit is the diagnosis and recommendation for treatment. You may hope for, "OK, nothing serious" or, even, "It's going around. You'll be OK in a couple of days." More usual is, "I'll write you a prescription. Take two of these a day and check back with me if you are not better in a week." The situation becomes more serious when your doctor suggests tests. Recommendations for hospitalization or surgery can be ominous. Let's examine a typical situation.

PROTAGONISTS: DR. WESLEY K. (INTERNIST), AGED FORTY-FIVE; MR. STANLEY V. (MACHINIST), AGED FIFTY-FIVE

Dr. K.: We're going to have to run some tests, Stan. I want you to report to the hospital outpatient lab tomorrow morning before nine.
Mr. V.: Why? What's wrong?

Dr. K.: *I'm not completely sure. I hear some things in your chest I want to know more about.*

Mr. V.: *You think I have lung cancer.*

Dr. K.: *Could be a lot of things. Remember, you came in reporting chest pains. You were worried, right?*

Mr. V.: *Yeah.*

Dr. K.: *Well, I don't see anything obvious. But something is going on. Maybe we can find out what it is and treat it early.*

Mr. V.: *But what is it?*

Dr. K.: *Stan, if I knew for sure, you wouldn't have to take the tests.*

Time may limit your doctor's opportunity to explain the details of each diagnostic procedure and disease. However an informed patient can ask questions and seek information in the public library. Some problems require discussion. For example, what happens when the only sensible conclusion to draw from a test is that another test is needed? What happens when the testing laboratory makes errors? It can be frightening to be called for a second set of pictures when you go for a chest X ray. You do not know whether something went wrong with the equipment the first time, or whether you have a serious condition that must be further defined.

Your doctor will try not to make a definite statement until it is warranted. Let's continue the story of Mr. V. and Dr. K. The commentary in the brackets will give you an insight into how doctors reason.

Dr. K.: *Well, now we have your tests back and we can consider some of the alternatives.*

[Comment: Doctors try to make decisions based on this is it/this is not it! Ruling something out means excluding a number of possibilities. In Stan's case the doctor ruled out heart trouble and lung trouble. The diabetes showed up in a standard blood test. The possibility that the patient was anxious because of changes in his physical condition could account for the chest pain.]

Mr. V.: Alternatives?

*Dr. K.: Yes, there are a few ways we can deal with this. For
one thing they indicate an abnormal sugar metabolism.
Some would call it mild diabetes. That may mean that
your condition can be treated with diet and exercise.
We can also add something to manage the amount of
sugar you have in your system. I don't think insulin
should be necessary.*

[Comment: Sometimes doctors appear to go against the "wisdom." Stan has learned that the treatment for diabetes is insulin. Dr. K. offers an alternative but Stan does not understand why. Dr. K. knows that it is desirable to manage diabetes by weight loss and diet, if possible, and chooses to try that first. He can use pills and insulin later, if necessary.]

Mr. V.: What are you saying? Are you saying I have diabetes?

Dr. K.: Yes.

[Comment. Diabetes is a complicated disease. Dr. K. can give Stan some pamphlets to read, but there is no guarantee Stan will read them or understand them, if he does. So Dr K. must say something now. The problem of what to say is serious. Some doctors have a canned speech; others try to adapt to the patient. The big problem is handling the questions that the patient *won't* ask.]

*Mr. V.: Well what's going to happen? Does that mean I am
going to go blind. I thought diabetes was incurable.*

*Dr. K.: Manageable. The future depends on you and how you
choose to live.*

[Comment: The question Stan won't ask is, "What's the difference between curable and manageable?" Dr. K. must explain the difference between an acute and curable disease (like strep throat) and a chronic and incurable, but manageable, disease (like diabetes). The explanation is complicated by the fact that "incurable" is not synonymous with "fatal," although Stan might construe it that way. Stan must learn that some diseases can be "managed," so they do no further harm to the patient. Diabetes is one of these diseases. So is hypertension (high blood pressure) and some some heart conditions. The problem of explanation is further complicated by the fact that diabetes, hypertension, coronary artery disease, blindness and infection are related. Doctor K. could give an extended lecture here, but if he did there would be several patients in the waiting room who would not get adequate time to consider their problems.]

Mr. V.: *But I came in with chest pains. What about the chest pains.*

Dr. K.: *I don't see anything Stan. Nothing apparently is wrong with your heart or lungs, but we'll keep watch. It could have been anxiety.*

[Comment: The chest pain remains a mystery. Dr. K. must remain alert because of the connection between diabetes and heart disease. He feels he is better off not bringing up that point now because it might make Stan anxious and create new problems. Dr. K. makes a note to keep checking.]

Bad news, not-so-bad news, good news. Most encounters between doctors and patients come out reasonably well. The doctor is able to find out what is wrong and recommend treatment. Some patients, however, may worry if the diagnosis is too simple. They may be responding to the medical encounter as portrayed on television and in the movies where virtually everyone has a horrible disease. But the human body is tough and, when cared for, serves us reasonably well for a long time. Actually, people usually feel OK most of the time. When they don't, something relatively simple is likely to be wrong. On the other hand, things go wrong, and doctors often must give bad news. Consider the following narrative of a perfectly ordinary trip June Smith takes to her physician.

Step 1. June Smith feels uneasy. Her friend has just been diagnosed as having breast cancer. June is forty. She hasn't had a physical examination for thirteen years, although she has been to the woman's clinic for her Pap smear once a year. She reads the magazines and is concerned about her health. Recently she has become aware of a vague pressure around her upper chest after eating. She has also been getting heartburn and has been using up three or four rolls of antacids a week. She decides to get an appointment.

Step 2. She calls Dr. Parker, the physician she saw thirteen years ago and learns that he has moved out of the city. The service tells her that his records are with Dr. Fletcher. Dr. Fletcher's receptionist tells her that Dr. Fletcher has the records and will be glad to send them to her doctor, but that Dr. Fletcher really cannot accommodate new patients. She postpones looking for a doctor.

Step 3. She wakes up one night with a terrible heartburn and a little regurgitation. She wakes her husband, discusses going to the emergency room, takes four antacids instead, and goes back to bed. In the morning her stomach is upset and she has a bad taste in her mouth. "Flu," her husband diagnoses. June grits her teeth and goes off to her job as an accountant. That morning, while at her desk at the title division of city hall, June Smith thumbs through the phone book and finds a doctor located a block from her work. "Anyone here know a Doctor Rubinstein," she asks the room at large. "Gus goes to him," Annie Richards says to her. "He's supposed to be a good guy."

Step 4. June calls Doctor Rubinstein and asks for an appointment. The person who answers the phone asks whether she is an old patient. When June says she is not but she is looking for a doctor, the receptionist explains Dr. Rubinstein's policy of beginning with a complete physical. June says that is OK but she is not feeling well now. "Is it an emergency?" the receptionist asks. "I don't think so," June answers, "but I am not feeling well and I am worried." The receptionist excuses herself and is back in a minute. "Can you come over at noon. Doctor will take some time off his lunch hour to check you out."

Step 5. When June appears, there are two people still sitting in the waiting room. "More time off his lunch hour," she thinks, but it turns out that one of the people waiting is taking her mother home after an examination and the other person waiting is the doctor's wife whose lunch hour will also be delayed. The doctor surprises her. She is in the office in five minutes.

Step 6. Dr. Rubinstein hands her a complicated form. "This is your report to me on your history. I want you to take this home and fill it out very carefully. We will get you an appointment for an initial physical in about a week, but I must have all the information on this questionnaire as accurately and completely as you can make it. Think through all the doctors you have been to, all the medicines you take, the things you buy at the drugstore, vitamins, everything. Where it asks for childhood diseases, check with your parents and brothers and sisters and get me all you can. If you decide to be my patient we will have to gather all your records." June is impressed by his thoroughness.

Step 7. "Now tell me what is bothering you," the doctor asks. "I have this feeling of stuffed pressure here, and a lot of heartburn." June points to the soft spot just below her breast bone. "When does it bother you more, sitting up, standing, or lying down?" "It bothers me a lot lying down. I used to nap after supper, but I can't because I start spitting up." "What do you do for it?" "I use a lot of (a popular antacid). "Well, at least it has no sodium in it," the doctor replies. Let me ask you some more questions." Dr. Rubinstein begins to take a medical history.

Step 8. Dr. Rubinstein has a hypothesis. June's responses make him suspect hiatal hernia, but it could be something considerably more serious. If there is a possibility of a serious disease, Dr. Rubinstein must rule it out. Meanwhile, June reports a long-standing love affair with baking soda. She says she avoids certain kinds of food and needs to sleep propped up on pillows.

Step 9. Dr. Rubinstein does a physical examination. He checks June's lungs and heart, takes her pulse and blood pressure, listens carefully to her stomach, and notes that she burps up as she lies down on the examining table. Maybe acid reflux is causing June's symptoms. Dr. Rubinstein is in the process of refining his diagnosis.

Step 10. "June," he says, "I think you probably have a condition called hiatal hernia." He explains what it is and what it does. June asks the usual questions. Is it common? Is it serious? Will I die from it? Do I need surgery? Dr. Rubinstein reassures her and then gives the not-so-good news, "I'd like to have some tests done to make sure we have nothing more serious going on there. You need to have an upper GI series (stomach X ray). I want to see if you have an ulcer in addition to a hiatal hernia." June expresses apprehension. "You mean you aren't sure what it is?" "I'm pretty sure, June. I've seen a lot of these. There is nothing unusual in your symptoms, but I always ask my patients to do this, just in case." Ahhh, those marvelous words, "just in case!" They are calculated to strike fear to the heart. But June covers up her apprehension. "What will it cost? Where do I go? When do I go?"

Step 11. Dr. Rubinstein's secretary makes the arrangements for June to get the tests. He also orders some simple tests of blood fats and proteins for basic physiological information about Ms. Smith. But there is a problem; the X rays are taken on Thursday morning. The radiologist reads them Thursday afternoon and sends them over to Dr. Rubinstein on Friday. By the time they get to his office, he is already at the hospital making rounds. He will not see them till Monday. June spends a bad weekend not knowing the results.

Step 12. The soonest an appointment could be arranged is Wednesday. Dr. Rubinstein has already called June to say there is nothing serious in the X rays, but there is a little something to talk about. A little something? June tries to manage her anxiety, but she really begins to flip when Dr. Rubinstein is forty-five minutes late to the appointment. He rushes in from the hospital winded, grabs the record, and begins to talk a mile a minute. There are seven patients in the waiting room, the phone is ringing, and his secretary has messages and questions. June wants her report unhurried. Says Doctor Rubinstein, "There is a hiatal hernia, a small bulge where a bit of stomach pushes through the diaphragm. Here, I have a pamphlet on it. Read it. It will tell you what to do." Dr. Rubinstein hands her a self-prepared mimeographed pamphlet entitled "You and Your Hiatal Hernia." "You said there was something else," June says. "Yes, a little patch over here." He shows her the X ray. "Look kid, you may be working on a little ulcer. We have to get you calmed down. Listen, it is too busy to talk now, can you make another appointment so we can discuss this calmly." This is a very decent thing for Dr. Rubinstein to do. He knows his frame of mind and he knows he has two intensive care patients at the hospital plus a newly diagnosed lung cancer victim sitting in the office. June's hiatal hernia is not the most serious thing in the world to him. It is to June, though.

Deadly disease lurks everywhere. It is hard for doctors to appear casual when they discover something seriously wrong. Most find it very hard to tell the whole sad story to their patients. Some even question whether this is desirable to do in every case. On the other hand, when the doctor advises hospitalization or surgery, explanation is absolutely necessary. Patients must give *informed* consent. This means the doctor must provide sufficient accurate information so the patient can make a decision.

The doctor assumes responsibility with each recommendation.

But it is the patient who must choose whether or not to follow the recommendations. Once doctor and patient have agreed on a course of action, the patient assumes responsibility for following instructions. The final link is feedback (the patient contacts the doctor and explains how things are working) and follow-up (the doctor recommends stopping treatment, continued treatment, or different treatment, depending on the circumstances).

A trip to the pharmacy. A prescription is the most frequent outcome of a medical visit. Most patients have learned that treatment comes in the form of a short note from physician to pharmacist. The process is not to be taken lightly.

Physicians and pharmacists have several reference books that list all of the drugs approved by the government (Food and Drug Administration). They explain the chemical composition of each drug, how it acts in the body, what conditions it is designed to treat, its performance record, contraindications (conditions that preclude use of the substance), possible side effects, what to do if a toxic dose is taken, and how the drug is to be administered. The book also includes pictures of the most frequently used drugs for identification purposes. Doctors are expected to keep up to date on available drugs. Publishers constantly update the drug information books with supplements or new editions making the most recent information available. Drug companies keep doctors informed by sending information and sometimes samples of new drugs when they are released.

The information about drugs is extensive and complicated, but what it adds up to is there are *no* drugs that have completely consistent effects on people. Your doctor must know how your body operates before he prescribes, and when he attempts a new drug, he must maintain continuous contact with you to be sure 1) that the drug is doing what it is supposed to do and 2) that it is not causing any side effects that are worse than the original condition the drug is supposed to alleviate.

You owe it to yourself to be properly informed about the use of prescription drugs. You must press your physician and pharmacist for complete information about when and how to take the medication, what it is supposed to do and how soon, and what the possible side effects are. Physicians sometimes assume you know more than you do and may gloss over important instructions. Pharmacists are often too rushed to do anything more than type instructions and glue them to the side of the container. Thus it is very important for you to be sure of the rules before starting on a course of treatment.

One of the best ways to evaluate the competency of your doctor is to pay attention to the way she prescribes medication. The oral instructions should be absolutely clear, and she should allow you time to ask questions about them. The doctor should not rely on the pharmacist to provide that information. She should have a complete record of all the drugs you are taking, regardless of whether they were prescribed by another doctor or bought over the counter in a drugstore in order to spare you considerable risk by advising you about drugs that, in combination, could have serious medical consequences. Some drugs must be taken with meals; others require a great deal of water; still others cannot be taken with particular types of food, milk products, for example.

When your doctor gives you a prescription, she is actually conducting an experiment with you as the sole subject. She is hypothesizing, based on what she knows about medicine in general and what she knows about you in particular, that a particular medication will have a specific effect. If things don't go as predicted, and sometimes if they do, she will want you to call back. An effective doctor will also provide the means for you to report regularly about how your prescribed drugs are working.

Life changes. Not all medical conditions can be managed with drugs alone. If you stop smoking, change your diet, go on an exercise program, or even change jobs, it can be more potent than penicillin. If you are allergic, you may choose between desensitization shots, modification of your diet, or specific treatment for symptoms. If you have serious conditions like diabetes or heart disease, it will be important for you to make major changes in the way you live.

When your doctor recommends you change your life-style, outside assistance such as support groups are sometimes useful. Alcoholics Anonymous, psychological counseling, and organizations like Weight Watchers can provide support for life-style changes. Conscientious doctors often rely on organizations like the

American Cancer Society or American Heart Association to provide useful information. They can also refer you to specialized support and information groups in which patients with similar problems band together to share information and learn about their illness. These groups help doctors motivate their patients to understand and follow treatment instructions.

Hospitalization: Surgery, Observation, and Therapy

Some conditions are so serious that hospitalization or surgery may be necessary. The hospital is used for three main purposes: 1) to diagnose, 2) to observe, 3) to perform surgery. In each case, patient consent is necessary. Except in cases of emergency involving an unconscious patient, no one is *sent* to the hospital. The doctor, customarily, offers the patient an explanation and the patient accepts or rejects the doctor's instructions. Once in the hospital, the patient must approve treatment at all times.

Your doctor does a great deal for you while you are in the hospital, although you may not see him do it. He monitors your condition, supervises the work of hospital personnel who provide your care, decides your diet, orders treatment and tests, and checks you personally at least once a day. Sometimes he consults with specialists on your behalf. Once you sign in to the hospital, your doctor is in complete charge. On the other hand, you have the right to sign out or ask to be transferred anytime you like. Hospital patients are not prisoners. A conscientious doctor will keep you informed about what is going on while you are in the hospital.

In most larger communities, doctors have privileges at more than one hospital and can offer patients a choice. If there is a choice, the doctor must explain the relative advantages of the hospital he recommends. You can ask whether the procedure he has in mind can be handled as an outpatient. Staying overnight is no longer necessary for some procedures that formerly required hospitalization. Even some surgery (e.g. hernia repairs) can be done on an outpatient basis. If surgery is recommended, you are entitled to a careful evaluation of the anticipated benefits and possible risks. Most third-party payment plans require a second opinion before payment for elective surgery is approved. Your doctor must be sure you understand his recommendation and reasons for it. Furthermore, you will need help obtaining and understanding a second opinion.

The process of getting a second opinion can be very delicate. If you seek a second opinion from among your doctor's immediate colleagues, you may doubt that the opinion is objective. On the other hand, if you go to a new doctor, you might have to go through the whole complex process of history, examination, and tests before you get the second opinion.

Your doctor spends many uncompensated hours in hospital committees and department meetings devoted to hospital policy, peer review, and planning. Hospitals are constantly monitored by the professional staff. In fact, hospitals are accredited by national organizations (J.C.A.H., Joint Commission on Accreditation of Hospitals, e.g.) that periodically conduct rigorous inspections of all aspects of hospital operation. You should avoid hospitals that do not have this accreditation. You should also be sure your personal physician is affiliated with accredited hospitals. It should raise some serious questions in your mind, if your physician is not affiliated with an accredited hospital.

Instruction and Prevention

Doctors can do more for patients than diagnose and treat. One of their most important functions is to instruct. Instruction includes not only information about your case, but also general information about staying healthy and maintaining a satisfactory quality of life. The case of Ken P. illustrates a typical response to a common condition.

KEN P. (STORE OWNER), AGED FORTY-FIVE

He started me on an oral insulin, or maybe it wasn't insulin it was something to get the sugar down. I didn't want to have the needles. It was always bad having needles shoved in my arm. In the army, I fainted when I got my shots. When the doctor said I would probably have to use insulin because the oral stuff wasn't working, I felt it was the end. I knew I could never learn to jab myself with the needle and I couldn't ask

*Angie to do it. I mean, she was a person who couldn't stand
the sight of blood, you know. Doctor T. put me in the hospital
and I stayed for a week. He said I would have to stay until the
dose was balanced and he found out I couldn't just take one
shot of long-lasting insulin, I had to do it three times a day.
After I got out of the hospital I didn't feel so sick any more, I
just couldn't even concentrate on feeling sick, I was in terror of
those three shots. About an hour before each shot, I got apprehensive. My heart would beat and I would think about jabbing
the needle into my stomach. I couldn't believe that the stomach
hurt less than the arm. I could go on about learning how to be
a diabetic. It's like becoming a new nationality or something,
or becoming a new species. Your whole life is changed.*

Ken P. might have found it easier to adjust to his condition, if
he understood his disease better. Ken did not understand that his
hospitalization was not for treatment but for instruction. His
doctor had to do research to discover how Ken's body operated,
how it reacted to various forms of insulin, what kind of diet would
be most welcome. During Ken's hospital stay, his doctor had to
teach him some of the complicated operations of the endocrine
system, the consequences of interference with their operation, and
how ordinary living could affect the system. He also had to teach
Ken how to care for himself. This included how to administer
insulin, how to plan a diet, how to respond to emergencies like
low and high blood sugar, how to manage exercise, how to treat
himself when he had another sickness, and how to include his
family in the treatment.

Patients must understand their personal responsibility in prevention and management of disease. Actually, the history of medicine is more distinguished by dramatic advances in prevention of
disease than in cures.

The smallpox vaccine alone prevented more death and disability
than all the medicines ever created. Vaccines now widely used for
measles, mumps, rubella (German measles) diphtheria, tetanus,
influenza and pneumonia, and polio, which we accept as a matter
of course, required great effort and collaboration from the scientific community, government, and even entire societies. The
only truly worldwide effort ever accomplished on earth by all

governments, and with which all governments agreed, was the WHO-(World Health Organization) sponsored eradication of smallpox.

The greatest medical advance of all times is the technology of sanitation that is directly responsible for greater longevity and better quality of life. Indoor plumbing and water purification prevent epidemics. Sewer systems, sanitary landfills, and control of toxic substances contribute greatly to good health. In American society, there is a great deal of information directed at people about their health and how to preserve it. Some of this information is very cogent and wise. Some is foolish and dangerous. The patient must also learn to be a discriminating consumer of information.

Patients can be trained to participate both in their own treatment and in the prevention of diseases. Ken P. had to learn how to administer his insulin. He also had to learn how to manage his diet so that he did not aggravate his condition. Many people could reduce their chances of acquiring cancer and heart disease, if they ate properly and exercised wisely. Research establishments constantly discover new treatments but all depend on patients' cooperation for success. Every doctor's effectiveness depends on patients who understand the possibilities of medical practice. Once a diagnosis is made and a treatment accepted, it is up to the patient to implement it. Only then can the doctor monitor the outcome.

Other types of medical support are popular in today's culture. Civic organizations sponsor blood pressure screening, blood sugar tests, cholesterol measurements, and sometimes even mass blood analysis. Kits are available to test for hidden blood in feces, to diagnose pregnancy early, to measure blood pressure at home, and to make periodic checks of blood sugar. The patient's personal medical arsenal is no longer limited to the thermometer.

Prevention

Most doctors urge prevention. They prefer not to have to see patients for conditions that did not have to arise at all. The following precautionary advisories represent main-line medical thinking.

Accidents. There is little doctors can do about severed spinal cords and smashed skulls. Conscientious doctors urge their patients to be careful at home, on the job, and particularly in vehicles. Accidents are the major cause of death or severe disability under age fifty. Prevention of accidents is easier than treatment of the consequences. For example, regular use of seat belts can prevent a great many serious injuries. The closest contact you regularly have with danger is driving to or from work. Working in safe conditions can also prevent terrible accidents. Some jobs have built-in hazards. For example, miners, woodworkers and chemical workers contact fumes and particles that predispose them to cancer, emphysema, or liver disease. Your doctor should remind you, periodically, to take simple precautions to protect yourself.

Genetic background. Your parents' medical histories can provide valuable information about your own physical condition. Heredity sets our limits and guides our capabilities. For example, if you know your parents had diabetes, high blood pressure, and heart disease, you can do a great deal to reduce your risk of having those conditions. If your doctor knows your family history, he can advise you how to live effectively within the range of your hereditary limitations.

Eating. Most of us have had a lot of bad advice on how to eat. Your doctor can help you avoid foods that might injure your body. Careful clinical studies show that avoiding excessive fat and sugar and consuming enough fiber (indigestible material) can help you prevent or control diseases like diabetes, high blood pressure, and some digestive disorders. Your doctor can advise on how to maintain proper nutrition.

BRENDA W., M.D. (FAMILY PRACTICE), AGED FORTY-ONE

It is very frustrating to have to try to teach grown people how to live. So many of their parents let their kids pig out on fast food and get started on artery clogging. They don't prepare balanced meals for them and they live their lives as if what they do has no possible consequences. Maybe I don't take enough time explaining, or maybe people are just too dense to understand, but so many of my patients are killing themselves. If I stay in practice here another ten years I know I will be seeing a

*lot of my patients who are my same age with some very serious
diseases because they are not careful enough about what they
eat. They never taught me in med school how to persuade people to change their lives and I really didn't know how important it was till I got into private practice.*

Food can preoccupy each waking moment. Athletes and runners
look for diets that will provide them with proper muscle tone and
energy. Slimness and attractiveness are now so closely associated
that a great proportion of Americans are on starvation diets from
time to time. This can become serious, for diseases like anorexia
nervosa and bulimia have become trendy among young women.
Excessive consumption of fast foods, salty snacks, cured meat, and
fats create potential hazards to the circulatory system. People who
eat fresh vegetables and fruits reduce their chances of getting colon
disease. A conscientious doctor is able to monitor what you eat
and advise you on diet and nutrition.

Toxins. Daily, each of us risks contamination from dusts, pes-
ticides, industrial chemicals, asbestos, formaldehyde, ultraviolet
light, and radiation. Recent discoveries associating sunburn with
skin cancer have modified the recreation habits of young sun
worshipers. The discovery that various agricultural chemicals can
poison people and that certain industries jeopardize their workers
with contaminants confront your doctor with an added responsibility to keep you informed. Conscientious doctors prefer their
patients to live in clean surroundings with unpolluted air and
water. Some young doctors are very selective about where they
locate their practices. Given a choice, they will stay away from
congested, polluted areas.

However, despite environmental dangers, most toxic chemicals
are taken voluntarily. Tobacco, alcohol, and "recreational" drugs
have probably caused more disease than the rest of the known
diseases combined. For example, your liver can tolerate alcohol
in small amounts but excessive drinking can do serious physical
and psychological damage. Tobacco is toxic at any level. Accidents
caused by people who are drunk, combined with the incredible
pressures alcoholism imposes on the alcoholic's loved ones, represent a problem of epidemic proportions.

Drugs are closely related to alcohol in their power to ravage lives. Conscientious doctors are not tolerant of these substances. A great many doctors gave up smoking when it was confirmed that tobacco was hazardous. Your doctor should be able to help you with advice and referral if you develop tobacco, alcohol, or drug dependencies.

JOHN D., M.D. (INTERNAL MEDICINE), AGED FORTY-FOUR

Many of my patients seem to want drug prescriptions not as remedies for particular physical conditions but as general solutions to life problems they are having. They may not be sleeping well or they may feel a lot of tension because of arguments with their wife or husband or kids or pressure on the job. Whatever it is, they believe I have a pill for it. Tranquilizers for tension, sleeping pills, pep pills, diet pills, stomach-calming pills, magic pills of all kind. Gilbert, of Gilbert and Sullivan fame, used to be captivated with magic pills. A lot of his librettos are based on people taking some magic pill and I swear my patients believe in that kind of magic. I must be very careful because I know my power to write a prescription is also the power to make a drug addict out of some unsuspecting patient who can't manage to cope with the way his life is going.

Tobacco is a toxin in any form at any level. It is even toxic to those who are not smoking it. Merely inhaling the smoke exhaled by the smokers around you can do serious damage to your health. Doctors sometimes appear to overstate the case against tobacco, but it was no accident that a great many doctors gave up smoking once the evidence of toxicity came in. The data about the effects of tobacco have been available for years but were ignored by the general public because the effects of tobacco are not immediate and the pleasure of smoking is.

Despite the fact that a great many people have stopped smoking and cigarette commercials are kept off television and radio, smoking remains a serious danger among young people and women. Lung cancer was formerly a disease that afflicted mostly men, but the number of male and female sufferers has become equal because of the increase in the number of women smokers. Equally unfortunate, in spite of the TV-radio ban on tobacco advertising, tobacco manufacturers have continued to seduce young people. The warnings on the packs seem to have little effect. Conscientious doctors try as hard as they can to convince their patients to quit smoking. Even though all people could reduce health risks by giving up smoking or not starting in the first place, people with high blood pressure and heart disorders must stop.

ELIZABETH Z., PH.D. (CLINICAL PSYCHOLOGIST), AGED
SIXTY-THREE

Doctors are sometimes much too flippant about telling people to give up smoking. They lose sight of how difficult it is to modify habits. If there was one thing I would recommend for all doctors it is to learn something about how to motivate people to change dangerous habits. You just can't say "stop smoking" and expect the person to be able to do it. You have to motivate them and check up on them and reward them when they do well. It is so very important. I have a lot of clients who come for help in giving up smoking and I think it is one of the toughest problems we psychologists have to deal with.

Physical fitness. Why all the fuss about exercise? Everyone seems involved; gyms and spas are springing up everywhere. For one thing, exercising is an excuse for young people with attractive bodies to put on revealing clothes and advertise themselves to the world. That, however, is not a sufficient reason to undergo the rigors of exercise. Doctors now urge people of all ages to exercise in a way appropriate to their physical condition. A conscientious doctor is the proper adviser for your exercise program.

Mental health. It is difficult to attain mental health, since hardly anyone knows what it is. Sigmund Freud said that sanity was understanding that you are about as unhappy as everyone else. Freud also defined pleasure as the absence of pain. Most of us are confronted with problems: bills, getting ahead on the job, being loved, doing something worthwhile in the world, having a happy family. At times we all feel overwhelmed by our problems and some of us feel miserable because we cannot solve them. The conscientious doctor is alert to these threats to mental health and your doctor should know enough about your life to take your emotional state into account when he considers your physical condition. Although he may not be qualified to treat your emotional disorders, he should be able to identify them and refer you to professional help when you need it.

RICHARD I., M.D. (PSYCHIATRIST), AGED FORTY-FIVE

I do all I can to cooperate with the medical doctors in my community. When a patient comes to me for help, I either check with her doctor for a medical report or refer her to a doctor for a complete exam. I wish the medics would give me the same courtesy. A lot of them try to treat mental illness and they don't know what they are treating. I know that if a person has a brain tumor I can't talk him out of it, but on the other hand, giving a depressed person a lot of drugs without providing other kinds of therapy will make him drug dependent and not help him improve. Psychiatrists and regular M.D.'s have to work together because the M.D.'s don't have the time or training to do a real job of psychotherapy.

Keeping Up with the Latest on Your Behalf

New medical knowledge proliferates at a rapid rate. Your doctor must keep up, or she will be of little use to you. Continuing medical education (CME) keeps her informed of recent advances in medicine. Medical school teaches only the basics of medicine. Your doctor must continue learning for the rest of her life. Medical knowledge moves forward so rapidly that most standard textbooks are obsolete the day they are published. Some medical textbooks have gone to loose-leaf format so they can be updated monthly. To remain competent, doctors must read daily just to stay up with recent developments. The basic science subjects, once thought to contain unchangeable facts, are also undergoing constant revision as new research becomes available.

Doctors are required to continue their medical education. Extensive continuing education is one sign of a competent doctor. While staying up to date is difficult, there are a number of supports provided for doctors to keep them posted. Pharmaceutical houses keep doctors constantly informed on new drugs and changes in details on old ones. Conferences are frequently held by various specialty organizations in order to keep doctors posted on current trends and innovations. Doctors often take time off for formal study at medical schools and specialty hospitals. Medical society meetings also provide enrichment by contact with other practitioners. Doctors often use these experiences as a way of exchanging information and soliciting advice from those with different backgrounds.

Journals are the major source of new knowledge. Physicians are taught how to read and evaluate medical research papers. Most medical journals are highly technical because they are written for the physician. Lay persons generally do not have the background to apply the information in them to their own cases. Recently, a major national television network has been providing a day of continuing medical education for physicians every Sunday. If you happen to monitor this network, you may be dismayed by the complexity of the information.

Motivation. Doctors like to work with highly motivated patients. The first step is knowing how. Aristotle once wrote, "the fool tells me his reasons, the wise man persuades me with my own." The conscientious doctor knows enough about his patients to tailor instructions to their personal needs. But Aristotle also identified two kinds of persuasion: artistic and inartistic. Artistic persuasion consists of explanations and good reasons. Inartistic persuasion includes threats and intimidation. Doctors use some of each kind of persuasion. A statement like, "you must take off fifty pounds or you are likely to drop dead," can have considerable motivational power for some. An explanation of the connection between weight, physical condition, and staying healthy would motivate others.

KEVIN G., M.D. (FAMILY PRACTICE), AGED FORTY-FOUR

I suggested Weight Watchers to a patient. Five weeks later, her weight was up five pounds. She said she went to the meetings. I can check that, but simply going does not do much good, and if she stops for pizza on the way home, it defeats the whole thing. I need to know what she is eating, and frankly, she can lie to me and probably does and worse than that, she lies to herself. If I can't get the truth I can't give good advice.

This is true with drugs, too. The PDR (Physicians Desk Reference) tells me how to prescribe drugs. I do it well. Many of the drugs we use are potentially dangerous. That's why they require doctor's supervision. I write out a prescription, the pharmacist puts the instructions on the label, and my patient still screws up. Antibiotics, for example, must be taken over a specified course of time because if they are stopped too early bacteria can adapt and grow stronger. Steroids (cortisone preparations) cannot be stopped abruptly, nor can certain high blood pressure medications. I need accurate information and many of my patients simply will not give it to me.

The most effective doctor is one who can combine instruction, diagnosis, and treatment persuasively. The doctor you choose must be competent and have a personality with which you are compatible. In this chapter we discussed what this kind of doctor can do for you. In the following chapter we will consider how to find a doctor who combines those qualities. We all also consider some major political and social issues than can affect your relationship with your doctor, and we will offer some advice about how to evaluate your doctor.

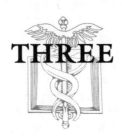

THREE

Evaluating Your Doctor

This chapter describes medical professionalism and how to recognize it. The practice of medicine is both a science and an art, with moral and political consequences for doctor-patient relationships. Even though many of these issues lie outside of the examining room, they can generate mutual suspicion and mistrust. By reviewing some of the major problems, you can decide whether you and your doctor disagree sufficiently to preclude a productive relationship.

How to Identify a Genuine Professional

A medical professional is, first and foremost, qualified. Qualification goes far beyond bedside manner. It is possible to get along well with a physician who is not qualified. Getting along well is not sufficient reason to use a doctor's services. You must be sure you select a genuine professional.

Medical schools and teaching hospitals try hard to sustain quality and to conserve the students they admit. In chapter 1, we described, the taxing and thorough training resident physicians receive in major hospitals. On the other hand, the system imposes such intense pressure that many young physicians enter practice fatigued and cynical. Some become excessively concerned with recouping the costs of their education; others may have been beaten insensitive to the needs of ordinary patients.

As a consumer of medical care, you must be alert to the possibility that your doctor is not competent interpersonally, despite qualifications and credentials. People change, and when those changes interfere with the care you receive, you may need to make the hard decisions to change doctors. Competency means the ability to apply knowledge and experience to your case in a way that satisfies your medical needs.

The first step in assessing your doctor's competency is to check credentials. Your doctor should have diplomas, certificates, and licenses displayed so you can check them. Furthermore, your doctor should give evidence of intellectual growth. Most physicians are active in medical societies and community medical activities. They take in-service courses, contribute to the training of other doctors, and maintain working and advising relationships with their colleagues. They are careful to maintain their membership on a hospital staff, for to lose hospital privileges is tantamount to losing their practice.

Most doctors belong to a hospital staff. New doctors in a community may occasionally be denied hospital affiliation because staff doctors, after a review of credentials and experience, may decide the applicant is not qualified or he represents a specialty that is not needed on the staff. All hospital's bylaws dictate that an intensive review of credentials be conducted to ensure that all staff members are fully qualified physicians. The typical review includes investigating whether the applicant physician has been involved in illegal acts, malpractice, or anything else that would make him an undesirable staff member. To maintain hospital privileges, physicians must undergo regular peer review. Any questionable case or allegation of malpractice is carefully investigated by committees established for that purpose. So, since the hospital is the professional hub of medical activity, it represents a major source of information about your physician's professional competence. If your physician does not have access to a hospital, he may not be able to serve you when you need him most.

Recent court decisions have challenged the right of physicians to maintain quality control over their peers. On the other hand, a number of journalists and consumer activists have attacked doctors for being too lenient on colleagues accused of negligence. Because this issue is presently so confused, it means you must select a doctor cautiously and continuously monitor his work.

Furthermore, medical training does not immunize doctors against the problems the rest of us experience. Most doctors live pressured lives. Their spouses often complain they do not spend enough time at home. Doctors have relatively high rates of divorce, suicide, alcoholism, and drug abuse. To paraphrase Gilbert and Sullivan, "a doctor's lot is not an happy one!"

These personal issues can have serious consequences for patients. An impaired doctor cannot practice medicine effectively. If a doctor's personal problems undermine his professional competence, it is the patient who suffers. As a patient, you should be alert to the possibility that your doctor, at any time, may have his professional attention distracted by problems that lie outside his practice. At that time, you owe it to yourself to change physicians.

Availability of Care

When you are sick you want medical care to be available. Many people do not receive medical service because either it is not available to them, they cannot afford it, or they choose not to use it.

People who live where there are few doctors are disadvantaged. Their doctors are often overloaded with patients and lack state-of-the-art equipment. Doctors gravitate to locations that have specialists, diagnostic facilities, laboratories, and first-class hospitals. The surplus of young medical school graduates have not gone to medically deprived areas. Instead, they have chosen advanced residencies in medical specialties. The net effect is those who can afford it have a wider variety of specialized, and often costly, medical services at their disposal, while many poor and rural people are still denied basic medical care. Programs designed to bring medical care to deprived communities have not worked well.

John K. (community activist), aged forty-eight

We worked for five years to get funds for a medical center in the valley. We are located sixty-five miles from the medical center. There is no doctor in a fifty mile radius of our town of 7,000 people. There are about 50,000 people in this valley who do not have access to a doctor. There is a doctor fifty-four miles south of here and several in the string of small suburbs south of the city, but they do not handle our people. Our people don't like to go to them. We wanted our own doctor so we fought the federal government to get some land from the national forest; we had community subscriptions and we finally built a medical center. That center has been standing now for two years. We got one doctor who came and stayed for three months. We give him free rent and we paid for one nurse, and he only stayed for three months. It has been two years now since we dedicated the center and we do not have a permanent doctor.

People who cannot afford medical care depend on public welfare and private charities. Neither government nor charity pays the full cost of medical service. Furthermore, government plans usually impose rigid controls on what doctors can do. Like other small businessmen, doctors resent the interference. Yet, virtually everyone who needs care can get it in some form, if they are informed about what is available and what they are entitled to. Most doctors do some eleemosynary work, but patients who cannot afford care may not be able to choose the doctor they want. Some doctors refuse assignment, both from Medicare and from private insurances. Others provide free care only to those who have been regular patients. Still others exercise their option to reject nonpaying patients.

Doctors can do nothing about people who reject their services. Communities can protect their citizens through mandatory vaccinations and quarantine regulations, but they cannot protect people from self-neglect. Many who reject medical service either mistrust doctors or advocate a medical substitute like Christian Science, macrobiotics, naturopathy, or faith healing. Some are simply afraid of doctors because of a bad experience in the past, horror stories they have heard from friends, or newspaper hype about malpractice. Whatever the reason, some sick people do not seek medical help. It is a matter of personal bigotry for which physicians cannot be blamed.

The Problem of Discrimination

Compatibility with your doctor can be affected by race, religion, age, and gender. The medical relationship is especially jeopardized by one-way or mutual lack of respect. Many women, for example, complain they feel patronized by their doctors, both male and female. Many blacks and ethnics feel uncomfortable with practitioners who do not understand their problems and their social style. Both language differences and cultural barriers can interfere with compatibility between doctor and patient.

The medical profession is disproportionately white and male. Why aren't there more ethnics and women practicing medicine? Do white male doctors discriminate against female or black patients? Are members of minority groups deprived of quality medical care? Is there any guarantee that one can get better medical care from a doctor who belongs to the same ethnic group? The questions cannot be answered in general. Patients must choose in their own interests.

Despite efforts at equal opportunity by medical schools, the number of blacks and Hispanics entering the medical profession is disproportionately low and has been steadily decreasing in the past three years. Women have not yet achieved parity in the medical process, although the number of female doctors has been steadily increasing.

Prejudice and social inertia account for these problems. Effective affirmative action programs have removed some of the barriers to qualified women and minority group members. Middle-class women have taken advantage of the new opportunities, though many qualified blacks and Hispanics are still barred for economic reasons. They simply cannot afford the tuition and cannot obtain the necessary loans. The result of this self-perpetuating disqualification is that the most competent members of minority groups are sought by virtually every profession.

The effects of residency. Most physicians are trained in major medical centers where there are a great many patients and a wide variety of diseases represented. The patients with whom residents work, however, have life-styles very different from those of their doctors. They may not be accustomed to medical care. They are often frightened and demanding and naturally suspicious of a situation where their lives are in the hands of stranger.

Hospitalization can be a fearful experience for those not familiar with it. The bustle and confusion in a major urban teaching hospital can thoroughly intimidate patients whose economic incapability denies them the opportunity to choose the kind of medical care with which they would be more comfortable. Sometimes being a patient in a major teaching hospital can be demeaning and embarrassing. Patients are constantly made subjects of demonstration. They are treated mostly by residents and are in absentia the constant subjects of lectures and discussion. They are seen by several physicians at regular hospital rounds, and they have little or no opportunity to form long term interpersonal relationships with their physicians. Despite the portrayal of the romance of the teaching hospital on prime time television, the fact is that teaching hospitals usually lack the personal touch, although the medical care provided is often very good.

For the young physician who leaves a teaching institution to practice in a middle class community, the contrast can be significant. In the first place, their patients will demand regular attention and empathy. Furthermore, their patients will be able to choose new doctors at will. The young physician has to learn human relations skills quickly if his practice is to thrive.

Women in medicine. The number of female doctors has increased steadily over the last decade. Projections made for the next decade indicate that parity in numbers will be achieved between male and female doctors. Once this happens, gender may well become an influential factor in choice of doctors. Sexual issues can confuse the medical transaction, and some patients prefer to make gender a major criterion in their choice of doctors.

Picture, if you will, a young college athlete faced with his first case of fungus infection of the scrotum (jock itch) who goes to the university health center and finds he must see a female physician. Jock itch does not pose a serious diagnostic or treatment problem. To the young man, however, displaying his genitals to a strange woman can be mortifying. A great many women are similarly embarrassed by contact with male physicians. The following statement illustrates some of the issues.

CORNELIA McK., PH.D. (PROFESSOR, WOMEN'S STUDIES),
AGED THIRTY-TWO

I am not prepared to accuse all of the male doctors in the world of being antifemale, but I have had a lot of reports from women about how doctors patronize them and treat them like children. They do not like being called by their first name, for example, while they have to call their doctor by his title. They also feel male doctors do not understand some of the problems that are special to being a woman. I think men are often patronized by doctors, too, and I think female doctors would have a hard time understanding some male problems, but women are particularly sensitive these days, and many times they will take unreasonable offense at things men do. On the other hand, some women are more comfortable with male physicians and are even uncomfortable with the nurse present during the exam.

I counsel women to be careful in selecting a doctor, and if they feel more comfortable with a woman doctor, they should choose one if they have the chance. They should also be sure of her credentials, though. Just because a doctor is a woman doesn't guarantee she is a good doctor. Furthermore, I tell them to be careful about leaving a very competent male doctor just because of some slight offense. Medical competency is what is important.

Religion. Religion can present doctors with some serious ethical problems. Some denominations have specific dogma relating to medical matters. Jehovah's Witnesses, for example, do not accept blood transfusions unless it is their own blood. Their religious convictions prevent them from accepting the blood of others.

There are a number of sects and denominations that oppose medical care altogether. It can be life-threatening when parents impose their beliefs on their minor children. Doctors are occasionally confronted with situations where, if they honor the parent's religious commitments, the life of a child can be jeopardized. If the doctor's ethics clash with parental religion, difficulties of immense proportion can arise.

Some religions require fasting as part of their religious observances. Such fasting can be hazardous to diabetics or patients with certain kinds of kidney diseases. Orthodox Jews often have restrictions on taking certain medications on the Sabbath or on major holidays. Some medications are permitted and others not. Doctors may have to take these religious considerations into account in devising a plan of treatment.

This issue of abortion has created considerable tension between some doctors and patients. Many doctors have been drawn into the controversy against their will. There is a medical procedure called abortion and currently, the law makes it available, under specified conditions, to those who seek it. The decision about abortion, as in all medical decisions, resides with the patient. Physicians must be careful to advise patients of the medical choices and to avoid propagandizing. Patients should not expect moral advice from their physicians, unless they honestly regard their physicians as qualified moral guides.

Aging. Aging is another issue that can materially affect medical treatment. Old people are more likely than young patients to have serious ailments. They can be fearful, suspicious, and exceedingly hard to deal with. They often require many drugs and long hospitalizations; thus their care is expensive in both money and time. Whether they are to receive special treatment by society is a matter for political resolution, but there is no question that they require special professional consideration.

It is not uncommon for older people to go to several doctors, each of whom provides a prescription. The possibility of dangerous drug synergies and overtreatment is very real. Furthermore, anyone can have difficulty remembering instructions about how to take a medication. The more prescriptions, the harder it is to manage the routines. Older people also present extensive histories usually involving many disorders and records with several physicians. It is difficult for physicians to accommodate to extensive detail. Older people have a special need to protect themselves by keeping their medical records accurate and up to date.

Both government and private agencies provide programs to facilitate good medical care for the elderly, though it is often physically difficult for them to obtain it. Getting to the doctor's office and understanding how programs like Medicare operate overwhelm too many senior citizens. Most serious of all, it is hard to find accurate information about available services. The physician should be a major information source for old people.

To complicate matters further, it is hard to anticipate the consequences of organized programs. When plans were made for Medicare, no one dreamed that the need would grow so large. Medicine has been able to prolong life, but unfortunately, a great many people whose lives were prolonged find it very difficult to pay for the sustained medical care they need to ensure its quality. Often, their medical expenses overtax their children, exhaust their funds, and finally place them in the arms of the welfare system. New proposals to ensure old people against catastrophic illness and guarantee the cost of nursing home care might alleviate this situation, but the issue of how to live out one's life with dignity and in reasonable comfort taxes the skill and morality of both the medical profession and society in general.

Change, from conception until death, characterizes the human condition. Everyone forgets that they, their friends, and even their doctors are constantly changing. The patient who has recently become physically or mentally incompetent is difficult for both relatives and physicians to accept and manage. Once-vigorous and alert physicians do succumb to age and life's problems. A good doctor-patient relationship adapts to these changes. This may mean changes in mode of treatment or life-style. It may sometimes mean changing doctors. These issues present the medical care system with serious problems that promise to become more grave as we near the turn of the century. The following statement offers perspective on the problem.

MELVIN O., M.D. (GERONTOLOGY), AGED SIXTY-SIX

To prepare for my retirement I took work in gerontology. When I was sixty, I took time off and took a residency in it. When I was sixty-two I moved out here and set up a practice. There are more than 10,000 retirees living in the immediate vicinity. There are a lot of doctors, but I am the only one specializing in the treatment of aging people. The most serious problem I have is keeping their records straight. When they move here they forget to take their medical records. Very often I have tried to get their records only to run into doctors who have died or retired, leaving the records unavailable. It is also hard for me to get them to keep me informed when they go to other doctors. Many of them are very lackadaisical, almost fatalistic, about their medical care, and they take dangerous risks with their health.

There are relatively few doctors, however, who specialize in problems of aging. This will become a more serious problem in the years ahead, when the elderly population will reach critical mass. Older people have to shop carefully for doctors who can empathize with problems particular to their age group and are willing to deal with associated problems of logistics and financing.

Dealing with death. Physicians deal with death all the time, but most will admit they still don't know quite how to handle it. It is not only a matter of dealing with survivors that presents a problem. A great many patients are becoming interested in planning ahead for their death. They count on their doctor to serve as their spokesperson at critical times. Doctors and patients are beginning to work together on issues like organ transplants and the manner of the patients' death.

If the doctor's job is to battle death, he invariably loses. No one has ever failed to die. Sudden, unexpected death makes both the physician and the family feel sad and helpless. There is little that can be said besides "I'm sorry." Sometimes an autopsy would help advance knowledge or is mandated by law. The doctor must solicit approval from the bereaved. Furthermore, every deceased person is a candidate for organ donation. The doctor must decide whether to solicit the family.

Organ transplants present knotty moral and scientific problems. British physicians have recently complained about removing organs from "brain dead" patients on the grounds that they are not yet dead. In America, some states have a Uniform Donor's Act that permits people to decide in advance whether they wish to be donors. For information, contact any major medical center in your state. Some states have made provision on the driver's license for you to indicate whether you want to be an organ donor. Keep your doctor informed of your wishes so that she can make appropriate decisions. Sometimes there are urgencies for a particular organ and doctors may be called upon to search for qualified donors.

Patients have the absolute right to make the decision about organ donations after their death. In the absence of a statement, their survivors may be confronted with the responsibility. Some people are morally opposed to donating their organs. Others feel that donating their organs for transplant is a final contribution to society. Whether to be a donor or not is the patient's decision but it ultimately involves his doctor.

Dealing with incurable disease drains the physician's emotional energy more than anything else. He must do what he can to alleviate the patient's pain, while dealing with family and loved ones. If the patient's pain is so bad that death might be seen as a blessing, the doctor must carry the news to the loved ones. Someone has to decide what measures to take. Should life supports be used, or should the doctor simply do all he can to relieve pain until the patient dies? Without instruction, the doctor must decide on the precedents of law rather than medicine. Euthanasia is illegal. Doctors may not arbitrarily discontinue life support systems, nor dare they risk denying treatment, lest they face lawsuits. Doctors need antemortem, specific instructions to make these decisions in accord with both the patient's wishes and the law.

Some patients take steps to prepare for their death. Many have wills that direct disposition of their property. A few have executed living wills to specify what is to be done about the use of extraordinary life-sustaining equipment and what to do with their body after death. While a living will is not always legally binding, it is a formal document that constitutes an agreement between you and your doctor regarding the conduct of your medical care in life-threatening emergencies and postmortem care when you cannot speak for yourself. The wise patient will discuss this with his or her doctor long before having to confront the issue. In fact, it is a good way for patients to discover something about their doctor's personal values. A physician who will not discuss these important issues may not be suitable for a continued relationship.

For patients interested in having a say about what happens in these critical and emotionally charged circumstances, we include a living will that you can examine. Read it carefully, for it makes clear the issues you have to resolve before you decide to be an organ donor. The living will (p. 72) is published with the permission of the Society for the Right to Die, 250 W. 57th St., New York, NY 10107. You may copy the form. If you do, *keep the signed original with your personal papers at home. Give signed copies to your doctors, family, and to your proxy.* Be sure to have your signature properly witnessed. You may even want to have the document notarized. For more information, you may contact the society.

Medical Costs

A solo medical practice is a small business. Your doctor has a payroll, pays rent and taxes, buys insurance, provides employee benefits, pays for utilities, amortizes expensive equipment, and disposes of expensive supplies. The humanitarian aspects of medical practice make it difficult for doctors to discuss finances with their patients, because it might lead some to believe their doctor is preoccupied with money to the detriment of their care. There is no question about the fact that the cost of medical care is increasing far more rapidly than other costs in our society. Part of this is because of advances in high-tech medicine, and part because of the urgency some doctors feel about recouping their financial losses. A good part of it, though, is because of increased demand for medical care resulting from the urgency patients feel to get the best treatment, whatever the cost.

Medical costs began to inflate when medical insurance became widely available. Once people discovered they could finance their

INSTRUCTIONS: Consult this column for help and guidance.

This declaration sets forth your directions regarding medical treatment.

You have the right to refuse treatment you do not want and you may request the care you do want.

You may list specific treatment you do *not* want. For example: cardiac resuscitation, mechanical respiration, artificial feeding/fluids by tubes. Otherwise, your general statement (*top right*) will stand for your wishes.

You may want to add instructions for care you *do* want—for example, pain medication; or that you prefer to die at home if possible.

If you want you can name someone to see that your wishes are carried out, but you do not have to do this.

Sign here and date in the presence of two adult witnesses who should also sign.

TO MY FAMILY, DOCTORS, AND ALL THOSE CONCERNED WITH MY CARE:

I, _____ being of sound mind, make this statement as a directive to be followed if I become unable to participate in decisions regarding my medical care. If I should be in an incurable or irreversible mental or physical condition with no reasonable expectation of recovery, I drect my attending physician to withhold or withdraw treatment that merely prolongs my dying. I further direct that treatment be limited to measures to keep me comfortable and to relieve pain.

These directions express my legal right to refuse treatment. Therefore I expect my family, doctors, and everyone concerned with my care to regard themselves as legally and morally bound to act in accord with my wishes, and in so doing to be free of any legal liability for having followed my directions.

I especially do not want _____
_____
_____
_____
_____
_____

Other instructions/comments _____
_____
_____
_____

PROXY DESIGNATION CLAUSE: Should I become unable to communicate my instructions as stated above, I designate the following person to act in my behalf.
Name _____
Address _____
If the person I have named above is unable to act in my behalf, I authorize the following person to do so.
Name _____
Address _____

Signed _____ Date _____
Witness _____
Witness _____

medical care through insurance policies, they began to make more use of medical services. As the insurance companies began to feel the pressure, new forms of financing like prepayment plans (HMO) and Preferred Provider plans (PPO) sprang up. These plans attempt to supplant regular health insurance with cheaper, more inclusive medical coverage. A recent and controversial trend is to have physicians supplement their income by selling prescription drugs. These kinds of innovations sew the seeds of doubt in patients' minds.

But there is always a paradox in the financing of medical care. Doctors provide a valuable service for which they are entitled to payment. On the other hand, the service is often provided to people when they are least able to withstand the cost. Many people fear being financially wiped out by medical costs, and media hypes about insurance policies designed to protect them against the failure of programs like Medicare feed their fears.

Financing medical care can impose a real barrier between doctors and patients. Conscientious doctors take care to make their fee and payment policies clear to you. They will also be attentive to your special problems. It is also important to remember how valuable medical care is when you need it. There is no price that can be put on a service that can ensure a sick child will not die, or a middle-aged person will have several more years of useful life. The issues of the economic status of physicians and the value of their service must continually be balanced. To a large extent, how well you and your doctor can work out these business matters will shape your satisfaction with the encounter.

Government and Medicine

The authors of this book believe that professional men and women ought to have the right to practice their profession according to their best wisdom, and that patients ought to have the right to choose which of those professionals to select when they need medical care. We also believe that medical care should be available to all, and sometimes this means the government must become involved to provide for the economically disadvantaged, to protect practitioners and their patients from scientific fraud,

and to see to it that important components of the research estab-
lishment are well funded. To the extent that government provides
an economic safety net, it must respect the dignity of aid recipients
and conserve the advantages of the free practice of medicine. In
more political realms of activity, the government should act to
restrain illegal acts and fraud and to support the advance of science.

The government has had a voice in medical practice for many
years. Federal concern about the state of medical education earlier
in this century set the stage for the Flexner Report that restructured
physician education in the United States. Today, federal funding
is crucial to the continued operation of medical schools and basic
medical research. The FDA (Food and Drug Administration),
which oversees the availability of drugs, is responsible for preventing the use of potentially dangerous drugs until they have
met the required tests of efficacy and safety. The National Institutes
of Health (NIH) plays an important role in sponsoring and co-
ordinating research. The Center for Disease Control (CDC) in
Atlanta is the most authoritative source of information for infectious disease in the entire world. All these agencies are funded
through the federal government. This is the "up" side of government involvement.

The downside is cost. Budget restraints impede many important
medical programs. For example, in order to slow down Medicare
expenditures and in blatant disregard of the changing population
structure (an increasing percentage of the population over time
is and will be over sixty-five), the federal government installed
cost restraints in the form of the DRG (diagnosis-related groups)
payment system. This procedure permits the government to set
hospital fees based on an average within a category of diagnosis
rather than permit the hospital to determine the charge based on
actual time and service given. The system was supposed to encourage hospitals to become more efficient and doctors to not
leave their patients in the hospital too long.

Like most programs with righteous purposes, some of the results were not anticipated. Early discharge, repeated hospitalizations, and considerable hospital and staff stress have been added
to an already overloaded public service. The medical arena is no
different from any other area of our life in which the government

becomes involved. If too much control is imposed, people lose contact with their doctors. Administrators can literally control the relationships patients have with physicians. The elderly and the poor stand to suffer most from reduced funding and cost-cutting regulations.

Some doctors have responded to government pressure by establishing their own bureaucracies. Private health service corporations provide a kind of medicine in which the emphasis is on services rendered rather than on doctor and patient collaboration. In these kinds of systems, the patient comes for service but has no claim on any particular doctor. The process reduces cost but creates some serious problems in continuity of treatment and maintenance of medical histories. The net effect of such collectivization is to reduce the influence doctors have on how medical care is given. Decisions about how patients should be treated must be made by trained physicians in the interests of good care, not by administrators primarily concerned with budget balancing.

Meeting Patient Needs

You have a right to expect your doctor to adapt to your individual needs. Such adaptation is essential to the continuing relationship that marks best medical care. Your doctor's professional competency, on the other hand, does not necessarily include interpersonal skills. There is little training available to doctors on how to conduct interpersonal relations. While some medical schools require courses in the humanities or provide minimal training in "bedside manner," most doctors learn to relate to others through experience. Furthermore, there is no generally approved style for medical relationships. Patients have different preferences; doctors have different personalities. Part of finding the doctor with whom you want a permanent relationship includes exploring for compatibility. Patients do have a right to be treated courteously by their physicians and with consideration for their uniqueness.

Time. There is an old saying that "doctors are born late." It is virtually impossible for any doctor to make precise estimates of how much time a patient will need. Some patients are sicker than the doctor anticipated; sometimes emergencies arise. Patients must take that into account as they sit waiting their turn.

DR. GUST M. (GYNECOLOGIST), AGED FIFTY-FOUR

I have been in private practice for nearly twenty-five years and I still can't get a day to come out right. I try to allot fifteen minutes per patient. The first patient comes in and takes ten minutes and I say, "wow, I'll get home in time for dinner to-night." False hopes. The second patient takes twenty minutes. The third patient takes thirty minutes. And so it goes. I stop scheduling appointments at 11:30 so I can get a half hour for lunch and I stop them at 4:30 so I can get out in time to get to the hospital before going home for dinner, but I rarely get time to go downtown for lunch and I rarely get out of the office before 5:30 or 5:45. Meanwhile, the patients get crankier and crankier as the afternoon wears on. I know there's nothing more boring than sitting around in a doctor's office.

There really is no contact you can have with your physician free from the pressure of time. While most doctors attempt to distribute their time fairly, sometimes you come out on the wrong end of the priorities and you end up waiting for an appointment, waiting to be seen, waiting for test results, waiting for a return phone call. Extra time given to one patient comes at the expense of another.

Doctors manage time pressures in various ways. Some simply refuse to take new patients when they are overloaded. In desperation, some doctors see patients on a first-come, first-served basis and avoid the pressure of appointed times altogether.

MARTHA T. (ALLERGIST), AGED THIRTY-THREE

I met a doctor who told me his idea was to charge by the minute. He thought he would get a timer, like a time clock, and when he came into the examining room he would hit the clock and then hit it as the patient walked out and charge two dollars a minute. A five-minute visit, look at the throat, write the prescription, ten dollars. A long consultation, a half hour, sixty dollars. It is an interesting notion. The patient gets all the time he is willing to pay for.

Would you put up with that?

Instruction. A medical treatment plan is really an explanation of alternatives from which you have the responsibility to choose. A conscientious doctor tries to explain the nature of your ailment and the differences between the treatment alternatives. Furthermore, she will regard each visit as an opportunity to teach you how to use the information he provides.

Your doctor should take charge during times of serious illness. If you are hospitalized or require surgery, your doctor will instruct you in what to expect, interpret information from specialists for you, and generally supervise the quality of your care. She will also help you learn to alter your life to accommodate to your illness. Cancer, heart disease, and similar serious problems require you to change lifelong habits to improve the quality of your life. Your doctor's support as you accommodate to these changes is very important. You will need her to check changes in the way you feel, monitor your condition, reassure you about side effects, and take action should something go wrong.

Your doctor will also teach you to use prescription drugs. A conscientious doctor will explain the dosage carefully and alert you to possible side effects. All drugs have side effects. Some are as mild as a rash or stomach upset, death is a possibility for people who are hypersensitive to a particular drug. Your doctor weighs the potential benefits of a drug against the probable risks and recommends a course of action. Drug reactions can usually be predicted, but some patients will react in unanticipated ways, depending on their sensitivity. Every drug marketed, including aspirin, has at some time in the past been responsible for such reactions and resulted in death. For this reason, conscientious doctors will not prescribe unnecessary medications and may seem excessively authoritarian in giving you instructions for those he does prescribe. Many doctors report their patients believe a visit to the doctor is incomplete, if they do not come away with a prescription. The conscientious doctor is alert to the possibilities of iatrogenic (doctor-induced) illness and takes care to protect you.

Courtesy. You have a right to expect courtesy from your doctor and her staff. You have no obligation to remain with a doctor whose interpersonal behavior you dislike. Between empathy and extraordinary unpleasantness, there is a wide range of personalities. If you do not like the interaction you are having with your doctor, reevaluate your relationship and consider alternatives. Sometimes you may have to accept a doctor with an unpleasant personality, if his skill and knowledge are important to you and there is no other alternative. Conscientious physicians will attempt to adapt their personalities to your needs. Competence and compatibility are the major criteria.

BROOKS G. (ADVERTISING EXECUTIVE), AGED FIFTY

When you are dissatisfied with your doctor you ought to tell him why. I tell my clients that they must find out why they lose business. When customers start leaving in droves you know something is going wrong and it doesn't help to cuss out the customers. Either someone is selling it cheaper or making it better for the same price. Or maybe they are treating the customers better. It's the same with doctors. I've been going to the same doctor for almost thirty years. A few years back he started having trouble at home; one of his kids dropped out of college and the doc was stressed about it and he started snapping at his patients. I told him, "Doc, I've been your patient for a long time and now I want my records because you just aren't a fit doctor any more." He stopped. He really cared. He asked me to explain what was going on and I gave him some free advice about merchandising and public relations—I guess you call it bedside manner and he paid me back with a complete physical and he really started paying attention to how he treated his patients. It may not work, but it can't hurt, if you want to change doctors anyway, to give your doctor a shot at shaping up by telling him what's bothering you about the way he treats you.

Doctor-patient contacts outside of the professional office are sometimes awkward. Doctors are apprehensive that people will raise inappropriate medical topics because they are held responsible for medical activities in and out of their offices. In addition, some people use social gatherings to show off how much they respect or detest the medical profession. They make doctors the objects of hostility or fawn all over them. Doctors want the same freedom to make their own social relationships as anyone else has.

It is sensible to avoid using office visits to discuss irrelevant topics with your doctor. You and your doctor need not see eye to eye politically or you may have major social differences, but there is no reason why these have to interfere with the medical relationship. While the conscientious doctor will try not to let his beliefs interfere with the medical relationship, sometimes valuable office time is wasted by doctors and patients discussing matters not related to their professional contact.

Personalization/depersonalization. Some doctors are affable and outgoing, others are detached and cool. Some doctors believe in laying on healing hands, others can hardly bear to touch their patients. Some doctors call you by your first name but insist on being called "doctor." (And some secretaries will refer to the doctor as "Doctor," e.g., "Doctor will see you now.") It is possible to become very irritated with the manner your doctor employs toward you.

Your doctor's personal style is crucial in making your choice. A recent study points out that people prefer doctors who are interpersonally close, can speak intelligibly, and treat patients as equals. Not all doctors can achieve the ideal. Your are entitled to seek the one you believe comes closest.

You may not have as much choice with specialists. You pay specialists for their knowledge and experience, and you may have to put up with personality quirks to get the information you need. Your personal physician should be able to mediate the encounter for you by interpreting the specialist's advice and overseeing the treatment. That is another reason why it is important to be personally compatible with your doctor. If you feel interpersonal problems interfere with the quality of communication between you and your doctor, make another choice.

Making an Informed Choice

Peer review. Every hospital, no matter what size, has committees to review each affiliated doctor regularly. These committees are made up of other doctors, the doctor's peers. Peer review is designed to guarantee high standards of medical care. It is the only effective method doctors have for ensuring in-hospital, high-quality medical care.

ARTHUR McC. (SURGEON), AGED FIFTY-SIX

I am chairman of our hospital review committee. I know there are incompetent doctors. I know there are doctors who make mistakes and I know there are doctors who take risks. I also know that most doctors prefer not to make mistakes and they try very hard not to take unnecessary risks. Peer pressure changes physician hospital behavior. Laws would not help eliminate incompetent practitioners, they would just clog up the courts with cases. What would help is patients choosing their doctors carefully. There is nothing that helps a doctor shape up faster than if his patients leave him. When the authors told me about this book, I told them they ought to make this point. There ought to be a scorecard for doctors for patients to fill out and if the doctor's score is too low, the patient should have no misgivings whatsoever about shopping for a new doctor.

You can be alert to the results of peer review by keeping track of your doctor's affiliations. If you find that he frequently changes hospitals for no apparent reason, or you learn he is denied hospital privileges, you should inquire why.

Quackery. Conscientious doctors also try to keep current on innovations and trends in medicine to keep you posted and counter the medical misinformation you get from the press or media. Your doctor should not be an advocate for untested treatments, nor should he be a purveyor of panaceas. You are entitled to a careful evaluation of the available scientific information for a new treatment, diagnostic technique, or whatever.

DR. ALBERTO P. (ONCOLOGY), AGED FORTY-FOUR

I had a patient once who wanted me to give him Laetrile. We hadn't even diagnosed cancer, but he had diagnosed him-

self and came up with a treatment. Sometimes patients ask for things they read about in magazines and I check and discover the story was premature or inaccurate. In fact, in our town, we had a nursery school director who was feeding ground up apricot pits to little children to prevent cancer.

When the information is proved inaccurate, it doesn't stop them. I have had patients go to Mexico for cancer treatments rather than try chemotherapy. They died, every one of them. I have had patients spend huge sums of money to go off to major clinics because they believed they knew more at the clinics than I did. They came back with the same information I gave them. I have chronic patients who keep finding tidbits of medical information about their own condition. Women read their magazines they buy at the supermarkets and learn about new cures that really aren't cures at all. Men read in their magazines how they can restore their virility or their hair. They come to me looking for the perfect prescription, and I simply do not have it to give. Sometimes I think I spend too much of my professional time trying to argue people out of some foolishness they read that was written by someone who didn't know what he was talking about. I keep up on my reading and I know foolishness when I hear it.

Home remedies and over-the-counter drugs are the first line of medical defense for most people. Some of them work, others don't. Self-treatment for trivial conditions like the common cold may not hurt, but serious medical conditions require specific treatment by an expert. They cannot be cured by over-the-counter remedies, megadoses of vitamins, incantations, or a shot of liquor.

Respectable-looking people with impressive-appearing credentials often appear on TV to offer remedies that can cause incalculable harm. The patient with cancer who falls into the hands of a medical quack can have diagnosis and treatment delayed until it is too late. Quacks argue that the whole medical profession is excessively profit-oriented or woefully out of touch with great scientific discoveries. They rely on gullibility and fear to bring them customers.

Quacks cannot cure. They exploit people for their money and endanger their lives. Virtually all alleged cures produced by nonmedical people have been proven ineffective and many are downright dangerous. Some popular diets, for example, are so unsound nutritionally, they take off weight by inducing sickness. Some recommendations for large doses of vitamins and mineral supplements can disturb your body's chemical balance and endanger your life. The conscientious doctor urges you to take personal responsibility for consumership in your selection of medical care. The Consumers Union (publishers of *Consumer Reports*) puts out a book called *Health Care Quackery* that offers sensible guidance.

But this does not mean your doctor should always go along with mainstream advice. The conscientious doctor keeps posted on innovations in diagnosis and treatment and may sometimes ask you to take a risk on your own behalf. If this is the case, then, he should be able to give you a complete explanation of why he is making the recommendation and what the possibilities are. The surest sign of medical quackery is the request to take a recommendation on blind faith.

The issue of malpractice. Doctors and patients, both, are concerned about malpractice. The cost of malpractice insurance is a steadily increasing factor in skyrocketing medical costs. Malpractice insurance costs are now so high that some doctors have actually been driven out of practice. For example, almost 20 percent of obstetricians, whose malpractice insurance premiums by the end of 1989 could run as high as $59,000 a year, have ceased practicing obstetrics and only do gynecology. Few new ones are entering. Both federal and state governments, however, are considering ways and means to bring insurance costs into reasonable control by imposing limits on jury awards and pleading procedures.

WILLIAM S. (CITY COUNCILMAN), AGED SIXTY-SIX

When the insurance companies canceled our insurance on the fire department and police department, we all got very worried. We contacted our Congressman and we demanded some federal help. We can't provide city services if we can't get insurance. Our city would be wiped out by a major lawsuit without the support of an insurance company. This raised the whole business of insurance in our minds. One of our councilman is a doctor. He says he can't deliver babies anymore because the in-

surance costs are too high. The public is going to have to think this through because a lot of their services depend on insurance in order to run well. City services and medical care are both at stake for all of us.

Malpractice is physician behavior that leads to a needlessly bad outcome. We all know of people who have, through no fault of their own, acquired diseases that result in suffering and death. No matter how good their medical care, it could not have saved them. Having a patient die does not mean the physician failed or committed malpractice.

Malpractice can be charged only when a physician gives less than standard care or makes a mistake because of gross negligence. Doctors have many alternatives from which to choose for any condition. But when a physician, for any reason, does not follow guidelines for standard care, or makes an error because of inattention or negligence, he or she is vulnerable to the charge of malpractice.

How can you identify malpractice? A bad outcome speaks for itself. But does a bad outcome of illness mean malpractice? No! It is malpractice only if the physician ignored standards of care or acted negligently. Doctors, themselves, may suspect malpractice by observing their colleagues in action. Often they use hospital reviews to pressure their colleagues to improve their practices. But disciplinary actions are not public information unless they occur in a courtroom. Hospital suspensions, censure by the medical society, revocation of license, and malpractice decisions are part of the record, nevertheless. Your best means for identifying a doctor who has been disciplined is to pay attention to the news and check for changes in their hospital privileges. If privileges have been revoked, you can assume the doctor's peers found inadequacies in professional behavior.

Only experts are competent to judge a physician's professional performance. You have the right to judge your doctor's actions with you. If your doctor recommends a treatment that does not make sense to you, discuss it or seek a second opinion. If you know something about how your body works, you will be in a better position to understand what your doctor tells you. If something serious has happened, and you are in doubt, seek a second opinion from an unrelated, unbiased physician. If reasonable doubt still remains, or you think malpractice has been committed, seek expert legal counsel.

Doctors are very sensitive to charges of malpractice. For one thing, it affects their practice. For another, most of them take pride in their profession. Contrary to past traditions, more and more doctors will criticize their colleagues in the proper forum. They will no longer protect each other. On the other hand, remember that medical practice is not an exact science. Doctors will disagree for good reasons. There are many "right" ways to deal with an illness. Keep in mind that you need not remain the patient of a doctor whose work does not satisfy you.

This book cannot settle the issue of malpractice. All professional groups, including physicians, have a few bad actors. Clearly, some doctors are incompetent because they have been poorly educated; some because they have let their skills decay, no longer care, or are overwhelmed by problems in their lives. Thus your initial choice of a personal physician should take into account the possibility of developed incompetence. Your experience should lead you to a wise decision. Your selection and retention of a personal physician is an issue of *caveat emptor*.

Nevertheless, your personal feelings are sometimes not a reliable guide. On occasion, you will have excellent medical results and still be angry with your doctor. At other times, you may be pleased with your doctor and have a bad outcome. The following issues are important to consider in evaluating your doctors professional competency.

Setting Your Standards

We have used the term, "conscientious doctor," throughout this chapter. A conscientious doctor is professionally competent to meet your medical needs and interpersonally competent to suit your personality. After a time, you and your doctor will write a record together. If you have seen your doctor several times and the diagnoses you received were generally accurate and the outcome of treatment generally good, there should be no reason for dissatisfaction. There are some aspects of professional practice to keep in mind throughout the relationship, but there is no official scorecard. You will have to decide, based on your own criteria, whether your doctor meets your standards. Each of following categories should play some role in your decision.

Your doctor's qualifications. Your doctor should be credentialed. This means he makes available diplomas, certificates of residency, and state licenses. Most doctors display these documents prominently. Graduation from a distinguished medical school does not guarantee competency, but it guarantees that the doctor has achieved a minimum standard of excellence at the start of his career. Evidence of residencies and fellowships, i.e., postdoctoral training, signifies experience and further supervised training. Hospital affiliations and society memberships are signs of peer acceptability. As patient, you should be suspicious when these indications are absent.

If your doctor claims a specialty, there ought to be evidence of that also. Occasionally, doctors claim to be specialists or confine their practice without having qualified formally. A specialist is a doctor who has spent three to five years in specialty training. If she successfully completes that training, she is then a qualified specialist in that area. Those who complete training receive a certificate. This doctor is now a board-qualified specialist. Look for that certificate!

If a doctor chooses, she may take voluntary exams to have a specialty board certify her. Passing the exam does not guarantee competency but it does indicate extra effort. In addition, the specialty societies offer honorary certificates or titles, if the doctor chooses to apply. These honorary certificates, called fellowships and masterships, are based on publications, community service, and contributions to medicine. They have nothing to do with clinical competency. If your physician does not display the usual certificates, you should ask her to document her professional ability to serve you.

Your doctor should also give evidence that she keeps up with innovations in her profession. You can ask about continuing education and check whether she suggests new treatments or is able to answer your questions about newsworthy events in medicine.

If you keep yourself informed, you will have a basis to check your physicians ability to remain professional informed.

The manner of practice. You must be satisfied with the way you are treated during professional contacts with your doctor. You are entitled to more than a silent examination and a prescription. Your doctor should explain the history taking and examination while they are going on. When he recommends a treatment, he should accompany his recommendation with an explanation of what you are to do, for what reason, and what the anticipated result is. Consider what he talks about and how he handles your conversation and questions. He should allow time for you to explain the nature of your complaint. The physical examination should include everything pertinent to that complaint as well as questions about related matters.

If your doctor prescribes medications, he should demonstrate he is aware that you may have seen other doctors and he should inquire about whether you are taking any over-the-counter medications. He should check your allergies and keep an up-to-date record of your drug sensitivities.

Reassurance is always comforting and useful, but simply telling you, "everything will be all right," is not sufficient. Information can often be more reassuring than consoling words. When you leave the doctor's office you should understand what he found out and what you should do about it. Recommendations should be explicit, whether they are for medication, more tests, referral to a specialist, hospitalization, or surgery. Above all, your doctor should offer you realistic expectations for recommended treatments. It is not helpful to be lulled into false complacency. Possible side effects should be discussed and any risks of treatment or examination should be explained thoroughly so you can give genuinely informed consent to everything done on your behalf.

Question everything! Your doctor should allow ample time for your questions and he should take them seriously. If you get the impression that your doctor thinks your questions are foolish or trivial, say so. In addition, your doctor should take time to instruct you about how to prevent disease and take care of yourself. This can (and probably should) include not only periodic warnings to use your seat belts and to avoid noxious substances like tobacco and recreational drugs but also advice on how to sustain good mental health.

Does your doctor seem to remember you? Some doctors appear to be very detached, responsive only to symptoms. Your doctor ought make you feel that you are being given individualized care. This includes addressing you courteously, not patronizingly, and at least acknowledging you, should you meet outside the office. Forming friendships with doctors happens like any other friendships. It takes time, effort, and sharing and is done completely apart from the doctor-patient relationships. Friendship and the doctor-patient relationship have nothing to do with each other. Do not expect your doctor to become your friend, although your new friend can be a doctor.

Evaluating office ambience. Even though sitting in a doctor's waiting room is not a recreational experience, your doctor should try to make it a comfortable one. The office should be pleasantly decorated, well lighted, comfortably furnished, with sufficient room for everyone who is waiting.

You have a right to expect the office staff to be courteous and informative. You should be able to get a prompt appointment and there should be an arrangement for phone contact so you can ask necessary questions. A conscientious doctor will arrange for someone to cover for him when he is on vacation or not on call.

Financial arrangements should be handled discreetly. There should be a fee schedule available to you on request, and you should know whether your doctor accepts assignment from your insurance company (or Medicare), whether he bills, or whether he wants payment at the time of the visit. Some doctors have their secretaries fill out insurance claim forms for their patients. Others provide a receipt suitable for including with the forms, if you have to fill them out. It is also wise to check with your doctor to find out how things would be handled if you were unable to pay for your medical care. If charges seem unreasonable, call around to other doctors and compare prices. Know what you are paying for!

What happens on a typical visit? There is no way to avoid some delay both in getting and in keeping appointments, but long waits may indicate your doctor is overloaded, disorganized, or possibly dealing with someone's complex illness. Once you see the doctor, insist on enough time to cover all your concerns. Spend your appointment explaining your complaints and asking questions.

You should be able to understand what the doctor says to you. If your doctor speaks only in technical medical terms and is not responsive to questions, you aren't getting enough clear information to assume responsibility for your portion of your own care. A prescription should include what it is for, how it is to be taken, and how often. Check also whether your doctor authorizes the pharmacist to give you generic drugs. This can save you considerable money. Finally, unlimited refills are rarely justified, especially on tranquilizers, sedatives, antidepressants and other drugs that may be potentially addictive or have serious side effects. Conscientious doctors urge their patients to stay in touch to see if they still need the medication or to report side effects.

If your doctor recommends tests, consultation with a specialist, hospitalization, or surgery, you have a right to a complete explanation. You should know the purpose of each recommended test and arrange to get results promptly.

The final component of an effective medical relationship is feedback. Be careful of doctors who do not respond promptly to phone calls or who seem unwilling to deal with you except during office visits. When you are being treated you need to keep contact open in case of side effects from medication or worsening symptoms. The conscientious doctor wants reports, even if the treatment is working.

Another way to evaluate your medical care is to examine emergency responses. Sometimes you perceive a condition as serious, and your doctor will tell you it is not. On the other hand, if you experience a genuine emergency, your doctor should be available, or he should have someone of equal skill immediately available. In emergency circumstances, your doctor's responsibility lies in providing immediate medical care, if not by himself, by others equally competent, until he arrives to take charge of your case.

Very few doctors will make house calls these days. They are rarely necessary. Furthermore, it is difficult to carry all the necessary equipment on a house call. On the other hand, it is sometimes very difficult to get to your doctor's office. In some large cities, physicians have formed groups that provide house calls for people who cannot expedite office visits. If you need such care, your personal physician ought to be able to explain your options.

Some patients prefer the convenience of going to a doctor who keeps diagnostic equipment in his office. Cardiograms, sigmoidoscopy, and other procedures are available in some offices. Some will also handle your immunization and allergy shots. If this is important to you, check in advance to be sure your doctor provides these and other services you want.

The bottom line. The following is a list of the essential elements of conscientious doctoring.

1. You should be able to get an appointment when you need it.
2. You should be able to get answers to your questions about symptoms, medications, and changes in your condition both in person and on the phone.
3. Your doctor should be properly qualified and affiliated with an accredited hospital.
4. Your doctor should have arrangements with other competent doctors to be available when he is off.
5. Your doctor's answering service should respond promptly and be able to reach your doctor or a substitute quickly.
6. Your doctor should provide necessary explanations in language you can understand about medication, treatment, tests, referral to specialists, recommended surgery, and hospitalization.
7. Your doctor should coordinate your medical care.
8. Your doctor should maintain complete, up-to-date records.
9. Your doctor should treat you with courtesy and civility.

Future Prospects: Prevention and Cure

The future of medicine holds both promises and problems. Most of us can look forward to long life and excellent medical care. As an informed user of medical care, you should keep posted on the news. Consult with your doctor about discoveries and innovations, when applicable to your problem.

Public health and prevention. The article "Waiting for Interferon" by Charles Fox in the September 1982 issue of *Harper's* describes the anguish of a young multiple sclerosis victim given false hope by media reports of a cure. Do not accept uncritically all you hear and read.

Significant medical breakthroughs are rare. Throughout history, the most spectacular medical advances have been in preventive medicine. Indoor plumbing probably saved more lives than any other scientific discovery. Vaccination and antibiotics have been major weapons in the war against serious infectious diseases. The government has consistently supported research for the purpose of discovering ways to cure and prevent disease. Recent breakthroughs in management and treatment of AIDS, for example, are the result of cooperation between government and private industry in the public interest.

But there is a considerable time gap between announcements of medical discoveries and their general availability. In the years ahead we will hear reports of advances against major killers like cancer, AIDS, and heart disease. But new diseases appear as old ones are controlled. For example, virulent forms of venereal disease, like Chlamydia and AIDS, have supplanted syphilis and gonorrhea.

Transplants and mechanical hearts have made headlines, but these have very little impact on the huge number of people who have heart disease. On the other hand, the recent discoveries that atherosclerosis (hardening of the arteries with cholesterol) can be reversed by careful attention to eating patterns and that stopping smoking prevents serious heart conditions give hope to both sufferers and potential sufferers. These findings are not dramatic cures. They demand careful physician supervision over a long period of time, as well as considerable cooperation and discipline on the part of the patients.

Dr. Karen B. (cardiology), aged forty-four

I have file cabinets full of diet sheets, exercise programs, and direction on how to give up smoking. I have leaflets from the federal government, Weight Watchers, the Heart Association, the Diabetes association, and U.S.D.A. I have made up my own direction sheets that I give to patients. When I diagnose heart disease, I try to explain to my patients what they can expect. I can't predict the future, of course, but the odds are with me when I tell them they can be helped if they stop smoking and change the way they eat. The problem is, there is no way for the patients to make a comparison. If they do things one way, they can't tell how it would have been, if they had done it another way. They can go on a diet and lose weight and feel pretty good, but there really is no way I can convince them that this wouldn't have happened had they stayed with their old ways of eating, or if they refuse to diet, they can always claim that dieting wouldn't have done any good anyway. And smokers have so many rationalizations for that lousy habit. I can't begin to tell you how angry I get when I see a patient smoking himself right into the grave. It is so stupid how many ways people can find to hurt themselves.

Progress against cancer is hard to assess. Although the total number of cases appears to remain constant, certain cancers (like Hodgkin's disease) have been brought under control. Convenient early detection devices help alert patients to get medical care when the prognosis is best. Colo-rectal cancer, for example, has always been difficult to deal with because patients have found it hard to talk about. Now, however, simple kits are available to check for occult (hidden) blood in the feces in the privacy of their homes.

Current dietary recommendations to prevent cancer and reverse atherosclerosis may not yet be proven, but based on the latest data, they are worth trying. Recommendations that people eat more fiber and fish while reducing consumption of cured meats and fats may prove quite useful. Citizen action against environmental causes of cancer may also be helpful in the long haul.

Cures for diseases like AIDS, Alzheimer's disease, muscular dystrophy, multiple sclerosis, and others, have not yet been found. There is still no cure for the common cold. Progress against disease demands cooperation between citizens, government, and private industry.

High-technology medicine. High-tech medicine saves lives. People who would have been dead ten years ago now survive with the aid of high-tech pumps, tubes, and computer-operated devices.

These marvelous, expensive devices create problems that never existed before. For example, sometimes people are sustained in a life with no quality. Some are brain dead, who, like Karen Ann Quinlan, though in a coma, can be kept alive almost indefinitely. High-technology medicine confronts both doctor and patient with the highly emotional question; under what circumstances should life be sustained.

The death in 1987, of the last surviving permanent mechanical heart patient, raises the question of the relative value of dramatic high-tech medicine. Virtually every doctor has been confronted at one time or another with a decision of whether or not to use heroic measures to keep a patient alive. These decisions impose great pressure. Most patients have not considered the possibility that they may be affected by such a decision and failed to inform their doctor about their preferences before they became ill.

One point of view argues that life should be sustained at all costs, since a cure could be found at any moment. The opposition argues that it is inhumane to sustain a person who is unconscious or suffering great pain beyond any chance of recovery. You and your doctor must collaborate in resolving these issues before they arise. Your doctor can carry out your wishes only if you make them clear.

Some high-tech advances promise great benefits to all. New diagnostic machines such as multichannel chemical analyzers, computerized axial tomography (CAT scanner), and ultrasound machines have become widely available. Every patient near a well-equipped community hospital now has access to the most advanced diagnostic methods. Ultrasound, for example, to assess the intra-uterine development of a child has been made compact enough to be available in an obstetrician's office. CAT-scanning permits examination of hidden areas of the body with minimum radiation risk. Likewise, a new scanning method called nuclear magnetic resonance imaging can use the body's own actions to create an image, without using X rays at all. New high tech procedures are more accurate and less invasive than those previously used.

These new procedures mean you can walk out of the doctor's office and know the results, rather than undergo the suspense of waiting while X rays are developed and read. Compare the risks and costs of arterial catheterization with new cardiological measurement devices. The colonoscope is considerably more accurate than X rays in discovering some intestinal diseases. You and your physician must consider cost, inconvenience, risk, and accuracy in deciding on diagnostic measures. When third-party payers cover the bill, high-tech is usually the first choice. For those with limited or no health insurance, the costs of high-tech medicine are too high. The individual health careprovider, however, cannot be expected to compensate for errors made by society and its legislatures.

Impending Changes in the Practice of Medicine

An informed consumer of medical care will be alert to changes in the way medicine is practiced. A number of trends appear likely to change the way doctors and patients relate to one other. Doctor oversupply, rising medical costs, and governmental involvement portend extensive changes in the medical milieu. Federal legislation is currently being prepared to provide insurance for catastrophic illness, while most states are moving ahead in provision of medical service to the economically deprived. The result has been a trend away from traditional private practice by a sizable minority of physicians into other forms of medical care delivery. You are likely to confront some new medical care choices in the near future.

Some physicians are becoming entrepreneurial. They combine their practices to cut overhead and facilitate consultation. Patients must be cautious about group practices to be sure their right to a personal physician is protected. Group medical practice synthesizes the services of medical specialists. There is an advantage to having a wide variety of experts readily available. On the other hand, moving from expert to expert dehumanizes your care. Without a personal physician to coordinate information, you may be bewildered. Specialists concentrate their attention on diseased *parts* of the body. Your personal physician helps you understand and apply the information. Normally, you are referred to a specialist by your doctor. You may not even see the specialist. Tests or X rays are taken and interpreted. Specialists are paid for particular knowledge useful in your case to be interpreted and applied by your physician. Without the services of a personal physician who knows you, the process can be dehumanizing.

Your personal physician can also coordinate the services of a wide range of practitioners. Dentistry and podiatry contribute to your good health. The specialty of "sports medicine" has recently responded to the trend toward more physical exercise. Psychiatry is widely available and great advances are being made in medical treatment of emotional disorders. Nurse practitioners and physicians' assistants were unheard of twenty years ago, but now they deliver much-needed health care where few doctors are available. Nurse midwives have released many obstetricians from the burden of routine deliveries and have made TLC once again a part of a normal delivery and postpartum care. In addition, special technologies now make it possible for people with very serious diseases to enjoy relatively normal lives. Kidney dialysis, portable oxygen equipment, and the work of specialists in rehabilitation medicine now make it possible for many people who would have otherwise been incapacitated to live outside of the hospital and in many cases, to be self-sufficient. Full-time rehabilitation centers specialize in preparing disabled people to carry on a normal existence. Occupational therapists, speech therapists, psychologists, and physical therapists combine their talents to support patients' recovery and rehabilitation efforts and help disabled people to return to the normal world. Finally, home health care specialists and hospices enable very sick patients to live and die in their own homes. This extensive menu of possibilities requires a coordinator—your personal physician.

The Issue of Empathy versus Science

DR. MERRILL B. (SURGEON), AGED SIXTY

I have been doing surgery for nearly thirty years and I had this experience the other day that put a whole new light on things. It was a simple case. A man on whom I had operated before came back to see me. His hernia had returned for the third time and he was wondering about whether a third opera-

tion would do any good. The records showed that the tissue was really nothing to get excited about the last time. Further surgery would have been quite difficult, involving the use of mesh and perhaps some tissue graft. The patient was overweight and largely sedentary. He wore a truss. I suggested that perhaps, given his life-style, he could manage without the surgery. He asked, "but what do I do about pissing?" I didn't understand the question. Then he explained that he couldn't bear down. Because of the hernia, he couldn't put pressure on his bladder so he couldn't void the way the rest of us do. He said that often, he has to hold the hernia, actually reduce it, while he voids, otherwise it takes him a very long time. He said this was OK in his own home, he could put up with it, but sometimes at a public urinal it was very embarrassing. He reported that he thought the truss would handle it, but it didn't quite because sometimes the hernia would sort of slip and he would still have to use his hand to control the pressure.

It occurred to me that I have very little ability to understand what my patients feel. I have been blessed. I have never had to have surgery. Here I have been cutting into people for all these years and I haven't the vaguest idea of what it feels like. I don't know what anesthesia is like, I don't know what it is like to wake up in the recovery room, I don't know what it feels like to have needles in my veins. I have been a very healthy doctor and I hope I don't have to find these things out from firsthand experience, but I will, no doubt, because I am growing old. And then, it will probably be too late for me to carry my new understanding into the service of the patients.

Doctors do not feel what you feel. They can only understand you by talking to you and examining you. This incredibly simple statement sums up the complexity of the medical transaction. Your doctor can never fully understand your anxiety and pain. You can never fully know the stresses your doctor experiences. A relationship characterized by experience and communication skill is the road to first-class medical care.

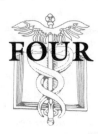

FOUR

Barriers to the
Crucial Collaboration

In 1985 and 1986 we surveyed 76 doctors and 475 patients. Our purpose was to discover major issues that interfered with an effective doctor-patient collaboration. Our sample was comprehensive and representative of the typical doctor-patient interaction. In addition, we corroborated our findings with several recent studies of doctor-patient interaction. (See the Appendix for the questionnaires we used.) This chapter summarizes the consensus of the attitudes of the doctors and patients we studied. It does not necessarily represent the opinion of the authors.

The Physician Respondents

The physicians in our survey were all in private practice, half affiliated with a major urban medical center with offices in suburban locations, half in private practice in a relatively affluent residential community with a full-service independent community hospital. There were twelve different specialties represented: general practice (19), internal medicine (15), family medicine (10), obstetrics/gynecology (5), cardiology (5), pulmonary (3), otorhinolaryngology, (3), surgery (4), urology (4), gastroenterology (3), endocrinology/immunology (3), rheumatology (2). Respondents filled out an extensive questionnaire that asked them about their attitudes toward patients and what they thought their patients attitudes were toward them.

In addition, forty volunteer physicians, twenty-two from the large city medical center group, and eighteen from the community sample responded to an open-end survey in which they described the characteristics and behavior of the "best," "worst," and "typical" patients they had had in the past year.

Many of the physicians were willing to elaborate on their responses. We conducted extensive conversations with nineteen physicians from the sample as well as with colleagues in medicine, sociology, communication studies, and other relevant areas. We also spoke with several of our patient respondents. We did not follow a formal protocol in these discussions. We asked our respondents to talk about what they chose, using the questionnaire as a source of topics. We asked some questions to clarify issues and circumstances. In most cases, what we had could be considered professional conversations. Our case reports were drawn from these conversations.

The Patient Respondents

Seventy-five adults were given a questionnaire identical to that given the doctors. In it they were asked to respond about their "personal doctor," "doctors in general," and "specialists." Fifty-five of our respondents were drawn from a list provided by the chamber of commerce in the community from which part of the doctor respondents were selected. Twenty were solicited by a class in research at a major university.

Our nonmedical respondents were 60 percent male, 40 percent female. They represented professional, white-collar, and blue-collar jobs. None were on welfare; all were covered by some form of medical insurance; thirty-eight by Blue Cross/Blue Shield. About one-fourth had a major medical policy with a deductible feature. The rest were covered by various per diem payment plans. About 5 percent were covered by Health Maintenance Organization or Preferred Provider plans.

Demographically they were mostly middle class Protestant and

Catholic adults between the ages of twenty-five and sixty-two. The lowest income reported was $22,000, the highest over $500,000, the median $31,000. If we lopped off the very highest and lowest incomes, the average was $36,000.

Each of our patient respondents reported some medical history. No one was in medical jeopardy, though thirty reported a chronic illness of some sort. Twenty-two reported problems like hypertension, diabetes, some form of coronary condition, chronic breathing problems, or arthritis. Fifteen reported having surgery within the past five years (mostly appendectomy, gall bladder, hernia, and hysterectomy). Five reported cancer surgery or treatment. Thirty-two reported nothing more serious than flu during the last five years. The sample reported an average of 4.1 doctor visits per year.

Our intent was to compare physicians' attitudes with attitudes expressed by the patients they were most likely to see in their offices. We avoided including people in our sample whose responses might be affected, either by inability to pay or by race, gender, age, or terminal illness

In a second survey, we compared two hundred patients who responded to a questionnaire about their medical worries and concerns while sitting in one of the authors' office waiting to be seen, with two hundred persons with similar demographics, who filled out the survey form in their home. The comparison sample was provided by a colleague in another city and was made up of people who had visited their doctor during the week preceding filling out the questionnaire.

Major Problem Categories

Linda's case illustrates the common disagreements patients have with their doctors.

LINDA W. (AUDITOR), AGED FIFTY-THREE

I've had trouble with arthritis all my life but all of a sudden, it really flared up. My hip was killing me and I had trouble walking. A friend suggested I go over to the university medical

center, but it was seventy-five miles away. It took a month to get an appointment with the specialist in town, so I got an appointment at the medical center. They kept me overnight and ran tests. The bill came to $1,500.00, they told me I had arthritis and recommended that I see the specialist in my home town. They made a formal referral, so he said he could see me in two weeks, but only on Wednesday morning. I told his girl I teach a class at the church on Wednesday morning and she said "Doctor only sees referral patients on Wednesday morning." I had to give in.

When I finally saw the doctor he seemed like a nice guy. He had read the reports from the medical center and he made some recommendations for treatment. I complained about his girl and he got mad and said she was not "his girl," she was his assistant. I said she was rude and he said it was her job to keep him protected so he could deal with his patients properly. I told him I wanted the maximum treatment. I couldn't take this pain. He said that in treating arthritis you start slow and I said I was sick of limping and he said he didn't do miracles and well . . . we didn't get along at all and I was stuck with him. He gave me a prescription, told me I wouldn't notice any effect for at least a week. Then he said I had to take some allergy tests because I might be allergic to aspirin. I said that no one ever told me that and he said there was no record that I was ever tested. These guys really take care of each other. He charged me $80.00 for the visit and then there was another $210.00 in allergy tests to find out I wasn't allergic to aspirin and the pharmacist told me the prescription he gave me was like aspirin, so it costs me $19.50 for a bottle of aspirin. Come on . . .

Our survey located six major disagreements between doctors and their patients.

1. *Patients do not understand the diagnosis the doctor offers them.* They are confused about possible consequences of their problem if left untreated or how, if treated, it might affect them. They become apprehensive when tests, hospitalization, or surgery is recommended. They report they do not really understand how to use prescription drugs. They rarely ask questions about these matters, even when encouraged to do so.

2. *Doctors and patients have different expectations for medical en-*

counters. Doctors agree that their abilities in treatment are limited, though they sometimes act omnipotent for "motivational" reasons. Patients often expect more than is possible. Doctors feel successful when they make an accurate diagnosis with a good prognosis for treatment. Patients are disappointed because their condition cannot be immediately relieved.

3. *Doctors and patients lose sight of their mutual need for one another.* Doctors and patients see each other stereotypically. Doctors often regard patients as uninformed and willfully resistant. Many patients see doctors as cold and authoritarian. These stereotypes make it difficult for both to adapt to their relationship. Doctors often overlook important emotional considerations while they concentrate on scientific diagnosis and treatment. Patients sometimes fail to follow good advice because they were not adequately persuaded or were actively denying their illness.

4. *Patients overreact to intangibles in the relationship with their doctors.* And doctors frequently overlook small, but important, matters of courtesy. Doctors' personal mannerisms can alienate patients and cause them to overlook the quality of medical care rendered. Some patients complained about being called by their first name. Others alluded to their doctor's "authoritarian" manner. Poor office ambience and time delays also impeded productive professional relationships.

5. *Lack of communication skill suitable to the situation is an important source of misunderstanding.* Doctors rely on a technical vocabulary and often do not provide information so it can be understood by patients. Patients are hampered in providing information when they do not have adequate language to describe what is wrong with them.

6. *Financial issues are important, especially the inability of the patient to understand why medical care costs so much.* Patients resent paying for medical service and stereotype doctors as excessively concerned with money. Physicians often purposely ignore the financial consequences of illness on their patients. Doctors are frustrated when patients use cost as a reason for rejecting a useful recommendation. Some prospective patients reject medical care entirely because of its cost. Some physicians reject patients because they cannot pay for services rendered.

The Consensus

Doctors and patients each formed homogeneous response groups. We found no patterns that indicated subgroups on either side. Major variables like medical specialty or years in practice did not differentiate doctors' attitudes. Variables like age, gender, or occupation did not appear to identify patients' attitudes. Immediacy of medical care also did not make a difference. The pattern of responses of patients waiting to be seen did not vary significantly from that of patients outside of the doctor's office.

Patients, in general, did not seem preoccupied with illness or perceptive about medical care. They resented illness, though, because it interfered with their pursuit of satisfaction and pleasure. Their concerns were largely personal: looking good, being loved by someone, dressing attractively, and doing useful work. Almost as important were enjoying life and having good friends. A minority reported mild concern about maintaining a good diet, staying healthy in general, and avoiding car accidents.

It was interesting to note that making money, observing religious beliefs, "being right with God," and getting good sex seemed to be of secondary importance, about equal to recreation and having fun with family and children. A minority of our respondents worried about whether they were getting enough money for the work they did or just keeping their job. Some were very concerned with keeping up their exercise programs, but few expressed concern with health matters like stopping smoking or weight reduction. However, the few people in our sample who had life-threatening problems (cancer, kidney or heart disease, and emphysema and related difficulties) or inconveniencing (crippling arthritis, serious diabetes) diseases seemed seriously concerned about their health.

We had hypothesized that people, generally, would not be preoccupied with medical concerns. One of the serious problems that doctors confront is reluctance by patients to make medical advice and therapeutic activity central in their lives. Healthy respondents were not concerned about prevention of disease. They expressed little concern about cancer, heart trouble, or AIDS. For that matter, they did not think much about other horrors like nuclear war or what would happen to their families after their death. They were only mildly concerned about the possibility of not having medical care available when they needed it or about the consequences of hospitalization. We concluded that our sample thought about medical care only when they were sick enough to need it.

We had earlier referred to Professor Hyde's conception of illness as a "break" in the continuity of life. Our data confirmed his formulation. The response patterns of patients, both in and out of the doctor's office, indicated that the relationship with their doctor was disoriented from the start because they resented the necessity to seek medical service. It is hard for a professional to be supportive and empathetic when he knows the client resents being there in the first place.

Best Patient, Worst Patient

Doctors had clear stereotypes about what they expected from patients. The profiles of best, worst, and typical patients showed great consistency. We had asked our respondents to anchor their answers by thinking of particular patients that represented best, worst and typical. Following are the consensus profiles.

The "best" patient. Best patients were from the same social class as the physicians. They respected the doctor's time, were good natured, compliant, and took their illness in perspective. They were polite to office and hospital personnel. The theme most frequently expressed was that best patients gave accurate information and seemed to understand what the doctor was saying to them. They did not expect too much from their doctors. Doctors did not agree on the nature of the disorder the best patient might have, nor about the outcome of the case, although half of the doctors mentioned their best patients died "a good death."

There is an important paradox here. West's (1985) findings indicated that doctors tended to block off patients' opportunity to ask questions. If doctors have high regard for the patient who understands, it would appear that they put themselves at a disadvantage by preventing patients from asking for needed information. Responses in the other categories indicated that doctors get a bit impatient at patients who ask questions.

The ordinary patient. The ordinary patient was either under thirty-five or over fifty-five. The younger patients had infections or temporary conditions like flu. Older patients were diabetics or had some kind of coronary disease. They sometimes talked about irrelevancies and were impatient about when symptoms would not disappear. They requested prescriptions and sometimes did not follow instructions about medication. They were occasionally disrespectful of office and hospital personnel. About 40 percent of the doctors reported this category of patient asked "too many questions."

Worst patients. Doctors regarded patients with serious terminal diseases as "worst" patients. Several qualified this with the statement that these were the hardest to deal with because it was difficult to confront a patient with a bad prognosis. Older patients, people who were unpleasant-looking, and people who complained consistently about their treatment also qualified as worst patients. Worst patients were often preoccupied with the size of the bill. Many respondents pointed out they felt it was inappropriate for their patients to talk with them about money. Financial matters were to be handled by office personnel. It was also interesting to note that most people in the worst-patient category either died or transferred to another doctor.

General physician attitudes. Our physician respondents were very concerned about time. Hospital-affiliated physicians consistently remarked about the pressure of seeing a great many cases with residents continually looking over their shoulders. Community physicians talked of the pressure they felt to see everyone who sought their services.

We discussed with some of our respondents the arguments offered by some researchers that argued doctors ought to give patients more time and be more communicative, humane, and sensitive to patient needs. Most agreed "in principle," but then pointed out that it would be impossible for them to take very much time to give patients sympathy and support. They pointed out that serious cases got all the time they needed. In fact, many respondents commented about patients with trivial complaints who put pressure on their daily schedules. Physicians must see people one after the other throughout the day in order to meet the demands for their services. Most of our respondents understood the paradox that if they give more time to each patient, they could see fewer patients. People who needed their services would be inconvenienced and those who received care would get higher bills. At this point, the conversations usually shifted to the economics of medicine, and every one of the doctors we interviewed called to our attention that they were not on salary and were required to see a specific number of patients each day in order to cover their overhead and make a living.

Though a great deal of scholarly literature holds doctors to be deficient in human relations, there is no consensus on the nature of the deficiency. Some of our patient respondents simplified the matter by saying they wanted courtesy and consideration. They complained that excessive brusqueness, authoritarian manner, and lack of communicativeness were characteristic of doctors they did not like. While few of our respondents accused their own doctors of being rude, a sizable majority believed that doctors in general showed little personal concern for their patients. This could mean one of two things—either that mutual respect developed over the long haul or that physicians were consistently cold in their dealings with patients but patients got used to it.

We raised this issue with some of our physician respondents who defended themselves by arguing that they were alert to a patient's psychological needs but had to focus their attention on medical matters. They understood they were not qualified to do psychological counseling and could make referrals, but they did not regard psychic treatment as part of the medical transaction. In short, most patients wanted sympathy, and most doctors produced reasons why they could not give it.

Our patient respondents were generally satisfied with their own doctors. Pettegrew confirmed our data by pointing out that 80 to 90 percent of patients felt their medical encounters were satisfactory. Furthermore, those patients who had a long-standing relationship with a physician expressed the greatest satisfaction. There are two ways to look at this. Patients and doctors learn to work well together when they have contact over a long period of time, or if a patient finds a doctor with whom he can work well, the relationship will last a long time. Respondents with little or no physician contact reported the greatest dissatisfaction. This could mean that patients stopped seeing doctors because they were unsatisfied, or that patients only become satisfied when they developed a productive relationship with a regular physician. The evidence was very strong on behalf of the conclusion that patients were most satisfied when they had established a long-term relationship with a doctor.

Economics and politics can combine to subvert the doctor-patient relationship. For example, it was predicted that the current oversupply of doctors would make medical care more generally available. Instead, young doctors took additional residencies and moved into specialities or affiliated with clinics. Our patient respondents were suspicious of clinics that denied them choice of doctors. They also preferred direct contact with their own doctors to referrals to specialists. In fact, specialists were objects of considerable suspicion. Patients could best utilize the services of specialists when their personal doctor served as ombudsman and information center.

Both patients and doctors were concerned about medical costs. Patients believed they could have lower costs without reduced quality of medical care. Doctors, on the other hand, were hostile to cost-control attempts. They argued that DRGs (diagnosis-related groups), which mandate consistent costs for similar procedures, resulted in inferior medical treatment. DRGs provided little leeway for individualized decision making, the doctors argued. While doctors and patients agreed costs were too high there was little agreement about any method designed to reduce costs.

Finally, we concluded, doctor personality was an important element in the effectiveness of medical care delivery. Some doctors simply are not effective with patients. In many cases, patients reported having a doctor they knew was competent, with whom they could not get along personally.

LANCE H., M.D. (EMERGENCY MEDICINE), AGED FORTY-FIVE

I discovered I couldn't handle the connection with my patients. I felt it when my patients died. I didn't know what to

*do for the families. Of course, there was nothing I could do
but I felt guilt anyway. I was frustrated when all the best treatments I could find didn't work. I couldn't handle it when I encountered a very sick patient who took up incredible amounts
of time but couldn't pay. I was in an emotional state all the
time and I wasn't making a living. So I went into emergency
room work because here, at least, I do the best I can and the
patient moves on to another doctor. I can be satisfied with my
job and not have to get myself emotionally involved.*

Patients did not understand some important features of the
doctor-patient relationship. For example, most did not seem to
be aware that they could change doctors anytime they chose. They
felt that once they had chosen a doctor they could not change.
Once they had shared a great deal of personal information, changing doctors seemed awkward and inconvenient. Thus a great many
patients continued with doctors with whom they were interpersonally incompatible.

Patients verbalized that they wanted quality care and a positive
relationship with their physicians. We discussed quality care in
the previous chapter. We will now draw on our data to describe
five basic problem areas in doctor-patient relationships: diagnosis
and treatment, communication, social status, financing, and ethical
differences. In the final chapter we will make recommendations
to patients about what they can do when they encounter each of
these problems.

Problems in Diagnosis and Treatment

People go to the doctor because they feel ill. They expect some
sort of examination, a diagnosis, and some recommendation like
a prescription or change of diet. Many doctors reported that their
patients expect to receive a prescription and are disappointed and
resentful when they do not get one. They rarely understand how
doctors do their work and thus may have unrealistic expectations
for what might happen. They are surprised when tests, surgery,
or hospitalization is recommended.

Patients reported a great many complaints about the standard routines involved in a medical visit. Among them were: the doctor did not let them talk enough, the doctor did not listen to what they said, they did not have an opportunity to ask questions, the doctor asked too many questions, the doctor was too impersonal, the doctor was too informal, the doctor did not wear a white coat, the doctor did not examine them enough, the doctor invaded their personal space during the examination, the doctor did not give sufficient explanations and instructions, the doctor talked in excessively technical language, the doctor was not sympathetic, and the doctor did not give them enough time.

These complaints indicated that the doctor's personal style is crucial to the medical relationship. However there was no agreement about what the personality of a good doctor should be. Each productive relationship between doctor and patient was worked out by experience over a period of time. Our data clearly showed that patients who had long-standing relationships with their doctors grew accustomed to the procedures and were satisfied with them. The question is, were patients with good relationships lucky enough to find a compatible doctor at the outset, or are productive relationships developed through mutual effort by doctor and patient? If the latter, is their any formula that can be taught to both doctors and patients to bring these kinds of relationships about? Our research indicated that, at the present time, there is none.

Prescribed drugs. Over half of the doctor respondents reported they wrote more prescriptions than they needed to. They ascribed it to patient pressure. Said one respondent, "I keep prewritten prescriptions for relatively harmless drugs to hand out like a pediatrician hands out lollipops, as a reward for being a good patient." Most were cautious about prescription writing. They felt that medications were ineffective and sometimes dangerous, unless patients understood how to use them and what results to expect. When a drug fails to work, the patient loses confidence in the doctor. Most doctors find it very difficult, however, to provide effective instructions.

DR. KENNETH L. (GENERAL PRACTICE), AGED FORTY-TWO

Most of what I see doesn't really warrant prescriptions.
There are a lot of ways to relieve the symptoms of a cold or the

flu or ordinary aches and pains. But the patients push me and when I don't prescribe they will invariably tell me about their friends and what other doctors do and I get the distinct impression that if I don't give them something I may start losing patients. I lose patience as it is with those who tell me about something they read about in Reader's Digest. Those popular magazines really practice medicine without a license and patients come in and demand something they read about. Often it either hasn't even been reported in the journals or it has nothing to do with their case, but try to tell them about it.

More than 90 percent of our physician-respondents agreed that the pharmacy is medicine's first line of offense. Two-thirds of the patients with regular doctors expressed confidence their own doctor does not misuse drugs, but three-fourths of patients believe doctors generally overprescribe. This presents a paradox: patients believe doctors overprescribe and doctors feel patients pressure them for prescriptions. Clearly misunderstanding about the use of prescription drugs affects most doctor-patient relationships. Patient sophistication would be useful. More firmness on the part of the doctors to resist patient demand for prescriptions would also help.

Surgery. Doctors are invariably surprised when their patients resist the idea of surgery. Surgeons prefer cooperative patients, but hardly anyone goes under the knife without considerable apprehension. Patient concern is exacerbated by the fact that doctors often disagree about whether surgery is necessary and, if so, what kind. Coronary bypass surgery is a good example.

CARL K. (HEART SURGEON), AGED FIFTY

I don't want to alarm anyone or reduce people's confidence in their doctors, but I am not sure about bypass surgery. I perform about one hundred bypass operations a year and I am perfectly confident about the need for most of them. But sometimes I think they give false hope. They may relieve the patient's symptoms for a while, but in most cases, they really do not reverse the process. Cardiologists sometimes send me patients because they think they have reached the limits of their skill, or perhaps, the patients won't cooperate with medical

treatment. But the bypass is very risky. We know how to per-
form them; we are actually amazingly skillful, but it is a risky
operation, painful, and patients often get depressed after them.
I am a surgeon and a professor of surgery and I must tell you
that it is a very serious matter to put the sharp edge of a scalpel
against the skin of a living human being. And I am also acutely
aware of anesthesia risks but I don't want to get into that now.

Some heart specialists recommend bypass surgery in almost
every serious case, others believe it is often performed unnecessarily. Estimates now indicate that by the turn of the century the
number of bypass operations will be reduced by 80 percent because
alternative forms of treatment are available. Patients simply cannot
adjudicate the pros and cons of most surgery. That is why informed
consent and second opinions are so important.

What makes it hard for patients is that they are unable to evaluate
the quality of arguments for and against surgery. When professionals disagree, patients become confused and lose confidence.
In any given case, an operation may be the only way to save life,
or there may be a great many medical alternatives. When the
patient has confidence in his personal doctor's recommendations,
the idea of surgery is somewhat easier to manage.

Half of the doctors we surveyed believed their colleagues recommended surgery too often, but that they did not. Patients were
in virtually unanimous agreement that surgery is recommended
too often. Yet, less than one-third of patients with a regular physician believed their own doctor would recommend unnecessary
surgery.

Physicians expressed considerable uncertainty about their own
recommendations. Several commented about how important it
was for informed consent to be genuinely informed, and most
relied heavily on second opinions. But getting second opinions
can sometimes be sticky. If the doctor who recommends the surgery suggests a colleague, there is a possibility of bias. A strange
doctor, however, might require an expensive work-up before making a recommendation. There is no easy way out on this one.

DR. GUSTAV D. (SURGEON), AGED FIFTY-ONE

There is no surgery that doesn't hurt. I'll tell you that I never
felt pain like when I had oral surgery on an impacted wisdom

tooth. The damn dentist had me under a local and he was dig-
ging around in my mouth like he was looking for the mother
lode. To this day, I don't know whether I needed that tooth
out. The dentist said "your tooth is impacted. It is lying over
on its side and it must come out," and like a jerk I never asked
him why. I mean, I should have said, "what will happen if I
don't have it out? Will I die? Will my lips fall off?"

So in my own practice, I look my patients squarely in the eye
and I say, "that gall bladder will have to come out" and they
don't blink an eye, right there, they say, "OK, Doc." So I say,
you should get a second opinion. Some do, most don't, but
when I try to explain why it should come out they get very
nervous and they don't listen to me. It's like they don't want to
think about gory details like will I be unconscious, will I bleed,
what are the odds that I'll die, will I feel better when it's done?
These are important questions and I think a surgeon should address them when he recommends surgery, but I swear they
don't want to listen to me and most of them won't ask. They
are just like I was with that oral surgery.

For patients, the decision for or against surgery represents a
major turning point in their lives.

CONSTANCE N. (PROFESSOR), AGED FORTY-SEVEN

*You can get very confused about surgery. I went to my fam-
ily doctor for my regular pap smear and when I called about
the results he told me something I didn't understand, he sort of
mumbled it and then said something about D & C or maybe
hysterectomy. He recommended a specialist and said he'd get
me an appointment. I got an appointment the next day and
that scared me. If it wasn't serious, why did I get an appointment the next day? Then the specialist acted as if I should
know what he was talking about. My field is medieval history. I
don't understand biology and even though I am female that
doesn't mean I know the names of all my internal parts. I kept
asking if I had cancer and he kept saying "no, but . . ." and I
really couldn't understand the "but's." So I went for a second
opinion. I found a lady OB/Gyn who checked me carefully and
then said all I needed was a D & C because I had some sort of
cyst or something. She was very casual in the recommendation.*

*So I asked what if I didn't have the operation and she said that
maybe if the conditions were right it could get cancerous and
to be on the safe side I should have it done. I went back to my
family doctor and he said he didn't want to get into the middle
of it. It had to be my choice, but I should do something. So I
asked the first specialist if he would do the D & C because he
was in my hometown and he said he would, and I asked if that
would take me out of danger and he said, so help me, this is
what he said, "maybe, for now . . ." Now how long is now? So
I asked, what if I had the big one, the hysterectomy and he
said, "might be a little more certain. Can't tell about cancer,
you know, creeps up on you. Have to keep looking." How
could I make up my mind?*

High-tech medicine. High-tech medicine has materially improved
the information gathering process in medical diagnosis but not
without risk and at considerable cost. X rays, for example, are
essential in diagnosis of a great many serious diseases, but they
can also put the patient at risk. Newer forms of diagnosis, nuclear
medicine, CAT-scans, and nuclear magnetic resonance imaging
may be less risky, but they still have an effect on the body and
are very costly. Procedures like heart catheterization or colonoscopy qualify as surgical procedures. They are invasive and potentially dangerous. That is why most complicated diagnostic
procedures require informed consent similar to that required for
surgery.

Most of our medical respondents reported that they do not
consider cost when they recommend procedures. On the other
hand, a great many also indicated they practiced "defensive medicine," that is, they used all available tests to protect themselves
against potential malpractice suits. What patients do not know is
that expensive tests sometimes give very little additional information. Informed consent includes understanding not only the
risks of the test but also its information value.

The doctor is the patient's main source of information about
technology. Often the issues are so complex that the patient must
rely on his physician's advice. When patients are unnecessarily
suspicious, it is hard to make an informed decision about complicated medical procedures. Half of our patient respondents be-

lieved their own doctors used expensive technology excessively, and 85 percent believed that doctors in general did so. On the other hand, our respondents expressed the feeling that they had no alternative but to accept their doctors' recommendations, despite personal misgivings.

Doctors reported a different problem. Two-thirds felt they could not keep up with technical innovations. They were constantly worried that they had overlooked some procedure or test that would help them be more confident of their own diagnoses.

DR. ALAN L. (INTERNAL MEDICINE), AGED FIFTY-THREE

I don't have time to read any more. Sometimes I think I get most of my medical information from the news broadcasts. I hear about things on the evening news and then I try to make a note to look it up and see what the facts are, but I forget. I keep up to date with the PDR but I really don't have time to look it over. The drug salesmen come in and hand me materials and I store them in a basket to look over but I don't have time. I take the continuing education things from time to time but it seems to go in one ear and out the other. These days I am tired, the patients are a blur. It is too bad. I could do better, but there just isn't any time. If it weren't for some of the bright new guys at the hospital, I probably wouldn't know anything new at all.

Patients find it hard to believe that their doctors could not be up to date. Two-thirds believed their own doctors were up to date in their medical knowledge, while less than half believed that doctors in general could fall behind in acquiring technical information. Patients also expressed their confidence that specialists were particularly well informed in their own fields. Nevertheless, keep in mind that there are over three thousand biological and medical journals that contain information potentially useful to a doctor. Furthermore, the articles in them are complicated and hard to understand. It is not difficult for a doctor to fall behind in his awareness of current procedures and treatments.

DR. CARL M. (UROLOGIST), AGED SIXTY

The longer I practice the less I know, it seems. I used to be able to make a diagnosis with a squeeze of a prostate and a glance through a microscope. But I have encountered so many tricks the human body plays that I am less sure today, even with all my experience, than I was when I first opened my practice. I think I need to ask a lot of questions about physiology and blood chemistry and I think I need to look at things inside before I decide whether to give a pill or cut in. I'll admit that the tests and stuff I ask for run up huge bills and often they don't tell me as much as I'd like to know, but I think it is better to be safe than sorry, you know. I don't want to take the responsibility for doing a patient in because there was a piece of information I could have gotten and didn't get. I think I even have a reputation for asking for too many tests, and some of my patients have asked me if I get a kickback from the labs, but here's the issue: I can treat or I can cut. Both are dangerous. For every procedure that can help there are possibilities that can kill. And I'd think it would be worth a lot of money to the patient to have me as sure as possible before I do anything at all.

What patients expect from their doctors is often unrealistic. A considerable amount of doctor-patient misunderstanding arises from patients' erroneous beliefs about their doctors' knowledge and competency and doctors' efforts to satisfy patient demands. If patients had more realistic expectations, it might reduce the aura of omnipotence that many doctors bring to the medical transaction.

Communication Problems

Recent studies (Katz, Cassell, West, e.g.) indict doctors for inept communication. They claim doctors are inconsiderate, authoritarian, perfunctory, unclear in explanations, and unwilling to deal with patients' questions. Our studies indicate that these charges are probably grossly exaggerated. Our respondents agreed that doctors and patients share responsibility for effective communication.

Doctors unanimously believed patients had the responsibility to provide information necessary for a proper diagnosis, while they were responsible for providing explanations and recommendations. Most doctors believed they allowed patients time to ask questions. What they did not take into account was the disparity in information between doctor and patients. A great many patients testified that they did not know enough to ask good questions.

History-taking and listening skills. Our medical respondents were confident that they listened carefully during history taking. Two-thirds of patients believed their own doctor paid attention to them during the process, but two-thirds also regarded other doctors as deficient in listening skills. Listening skill seems to be a common criterion of a good doctor. Unfortunately, there is no way to measure listening competency. It is easy to confuse the appearance of listening with listening itself. Furthermore, there are no proven programs for teaching listening skills.

Doctors were often critical of their history-taking skills. Half reported they sometimes overlooked important information or did not time questions properly to get the most reliable information. Two-thirds believed they rarely had time to take an adequate history. When a patient comes in with a serious ailment the pressure to act is usually too great to permit taking a complete history. Patients with chronic ailments, on the other hand, build up histories over time.

All of our doctor respondents reported many patients were either unwilling or unable to provide accurate and complete information for the history. Some patients are embarrassed by topics like elimination and sex. Many do not have language with which they feel comfortable discussing these issues. Most doctor respondents reported many of their patients willfully withheld important information such as other medical contacts and drugs taken. Patients, they believed, were especially reticent about reporting over-the-counter and illicit drugs and were often inaccurate reporting prescriptions given by other doctors.

Several doctors argued, during interviews, that patient failure to report drugs being used was especially dangerous, because of possible drug interactions. Several mentioned how important it is for patients to report medications given them by dentists, chiropodists, and other practitioners.

Most doctors understand medical language is often too technical, but they are uncertain about how to adapt to their patients.

Many see the alternative to be the use of vulgar language, which patients may find offensive. The result is many patients come away from a doctor visit unsatisfied because they did not get all the information they needed. Still, most patients understood that it was their own lack of sophistication that kept them from asking questions. Several reported they did not even think of the questions until after they left the doctor's office. Others claimed they knew what to ask but didn't know how to phrase it. It appeared that most potential patients do not know enough about their own physiology to carry on an intelligent professional conversation with their doctors.

Doctors were critical of their own recordkeeping. Three-fourths doubted whether they recorded all important information. Half believed their patients lacked confidence in the records. Seventy percent of patients expressed similar suspicions of doctors in general, though an equal proportion believed their personal doctors kept accurate records.

DR. FRED O'C. (INTERNAL MEDICINE), AGED FORTY-SEVEN

Ever since I opened my practice I have been trying to figure out a way to store all the information I get from patients in some kind of system that enables me to get at it when I need it. I used to write the notes in the record by hand. This took too long and I'd forget before I got it all down. Then I tried a tape recorder and had my secretary transcribe the notes, and sometimes she'd mess up some words so badly I couldn't figure out what I meant. And I was never sure I picked up the right stuff. It's easy enough to keep measurement records. Blood pressure, temperature, respiration, and like that and to check off what you looked at and what you prescribed. But it is the little things about how the patient looked and acted and some of the things they said that are really important and I am never sure that I made the right choices about what to keep.

Communicating advice and directions. Doctors are generally dissatisfied with their ability to give information. Three-fourths believed they do not give enough information to patients about prescriptions. They relied heavily on the pharmacist's instructions for backup. Nearly two-thirds of the patients report they have been confused by instructions given them by their own doctor, and three-fourths claim doctors are generally inept in giving information about medications. In a situation of mutual blame, patients ought to be especially alert about getting specific instructions for the use of medications.

DR. CURTIS McQ. (INTERNAL MEDICINE), AGED FORTY-FOUR

Mrs. D. has asthma. It was getting worse. I said to her," continue on your theophylline and use the inhaler four times a day." She said, "why do I have to increase the theophylline?" "No," I said, "it's three squirts on the inhaler four times a day, that's breakfast, lunch, dinner, and bedtime." There was a pause and we talked about something else and then she said, "I thought I had to take the theophylline three times a day. Why do I have to take four pills?" I wrote out the instructions for her. Sure enough, two hours later, I got a phone call from her. "Would you review what I am supposed to do with the pills and the inhaler. Which is it I take three times a day, which four times and which . . ." Well, it was confusing, but you'd think that in the management of a condition that concerns her so much she would try a little harder to understand what should go on, especially when it was written out for her.

Furthermore, patients have a tendency to distort information in ways that lead them to expect more than their prescriptions can deliver.

ARTHUR H. (MACHINIST), AGED THIRTY-FOUR

I took the prescription to the drugstore and I was surprised because it was a pill. I thought the doctor was going to give me some ointment for my sore muscles. I used (Product Name) every other time I had a sore muscle, so I couldn't understand why the pill, so I took the pill and I took them for a day or two and nothing helped, so I went and got a tube of (Product Name) and rubbed it in like I used to, and it took nearly a week for the pain to go away. I told the doctor about it and he asked me how long I took the pills, did I use them all up, and I told him I just took them for a day or two, and he got angry and said he said I should use them all up but if I did that it would have taken just as long as when I used (Product Name).

AARON W. (PHARMACIST), AGED SIXTY

I am a basic information source for most of my customers. I've had the store for years and I know most of my customers. I keep records for them. If they bring me all their prescriptions I can tell them when they have dangerous combinations of drugs. I am amazed all the time about how many of my customers go to several doctors and never tell the doctors they are doing it. One customer I know had four different doctors giving her tranquilizers. I can do some good here, because when one of the doctors calls in a prescription I can tell him what the other prescriptions are. I am not sure this is ethical, but I do it because I think the doctor must have the information. Also, patients ask me a lot about instructions and I try to type them out clearly on the small labels on the bottles, and then we talk about it and sometimes I have to tell them not to take this with milk and to take this on an empty stomach because the doctor forgot. See, nothing like a good pharmacist to make a doctor look good and a patient happy, right?

Most patients reported they have, on occasion, been disappointed with their doctors because of time it took before they felt better. Most doctors reported that a sizable number of patients complained to them that prescriptions took too long to work. On the other hand, doctors often do not make it clear to their patients what to expect. They are cautious about setting time limits because they understand the variability in the way drugs work. They also tend to avoid describing side effects for fear of iatrogenesis. This occasionally leads them to underinstruct their patients.

Mutual confidence. Mutual confidence is the essence of quality communication between doctors and patients. Nearly half of the doctor respondents reported they sometimes distorted information they gave their patients. They argued that if they told the whole truth, the patient might be upset. Patients, on the other hand, were unanimous in the belief that doctors told the whole truth.

The term "bedside manner" has been used to refer to the doctor's interpersonal skill. A great many patients estimate their doctor's quality by his bedside manner. For a great many patients, the ability to achieve a supportive relationship with the doctor overshadows professional competence. Although both qualities are desirable, it is easier for the patient to evaluate interpersonal skill (a matter of preference) than professional competence.

More than 40 percent of our respondents complained that their own doctor sometimes saw them as just a "case" not as a person, and nearly three-fourths believed that specialists dealt primarily with "cases." But the doctors nearly unanimously supported the statement, "doctors treat people, not diseases." Most doctors sincerely believed they were considerate of their patients' needs. Many expressed bewilderment and anger at accusations that they are insensitive or inept at communication. They do not know what or how to change.

This is an important proposition, in light of current assaults on the medical profession by the media and various researchers. It may well be that there are inadequacies in the way medicine is being practiced, but the assertion that "humane treatment" or "personal consideration" is needed begs the question. For one thing, there is no evidence that a particular manner of treatment is connected with a salubrious outcome. Nice-guy doctors sometimes lose patients, and hard cases sometimes win. Furthermore, humanity is a personal judgment made by patients. We talked to several of our patient respondents about it. There simply was no agreement about what personal qualities they preferred in their doctor.

Our findings indicate a high degree of satisfaction with medical care on the part of people who have developed a relationship with a personal doctor. Most dissatisfaction seems to come from first-time patients, patients who see doctors occasionally, or patients who seek care at HMO clinics and other facilities where it is not possible to develop a relationship. This state of affairs may suggest some changes that can be made by patients and administrators in the direction of developing long term medical relationships. *It may well be that no first-time medical encounter is entirely satisfactory to either doctor or patient, nor can it be, by its very nature.*

Two-thirds of the doctors reported their most important task was to fit their patient into a generalization about a disease or condition. This procedure may be bewildering or offensive to some patients, because it requires some detachment. The doctor may be required to prescribe for an individual, but he must rely on general propositions about diseases and their treatment to figure out his alternatives. The requirement for careful history taking and often detailed examination can interfere with interpersonal warmth. Patients who know this have less trouble with the process and find more opportunities to develop relationships with their doctors.

What is more important is that three-fourths of the doctors surveyed reported they had to detach themselves emotionally from their patients in order to cope with tension involved in dealing with sick people. Most patients expected some detachment, though half reported even their own doctors were too distant some of the time. Doctors confirmed this feeling when more than half of them reported they had trouble remembering their patients' names. They relied on their records, already indicted as dubious, to carry them through. Three-fourths of the doctors expected their patients to recognize that their coolness and detachment is a professional requirement and that personal involvement may get in the way of treatment. The issue here seems to be one of expectations. The more patients understood about how doctors did their jobs, the more tolerant they were of the "medical" demeanor. On the other hand, a number of patient respondents reported cases of arrogance and patronization that they believed were intolerable.

Excessive preoccupation with the patient's emotions can distract the doctor from applying the scientific method.

1. Evidence is derived from observation, examination, history, and test to document the existence of a "disease" or abnormal condition. This requires attention to detail about the patient. Preoccupation with patient personality can interfere with accurate observation.

2. The doctor must choose whether to treat symptoms of a diseases, its causes, or both, while taking into account the unique nature of each patient's responses. At this point in the process, the patient's unique history becomes very important.

3. Once the doctor fits a set of symptoms into a category, there are alternatives to recommend. The alternatives are drawn from generalizations and must be synthesized into what is known about the patient's unique physiology and medical experience.

4. Responses must be recorded so that the doctor can judge patient's progress. The patient's record provides a set of generalizations about the patient. The ultimate medical transaction is synthesizing physiological generalizations with generalizations about the patient's physiology. The process of diagnosis minimizes the importance of affection and warmth. On the other hand, motivation to follow a prescribed course of treatment requires considerable personalization. There is clearly a mutual burden here for doctors to be more considerate of individual patient needs and for patients to become more intelligent consumers of medical advice.

Political and social issues. There are a number of political and social issues on which doctors and patients seem to disagree. Among the complaints registered against doctors are that they discriminate against certain kinds of patients (women, the elderly, and the poor). These issues are not intrinsic to the doctor-patient relationship, but they sometimes muddy the water. For example, more than half of the patients surveyed believed that doctors do not give good care to charity patients. One-fourth of the doctors agreed, and most expected their patients to indict them on this score.

The description of the "best patient" given by doctors indicate they tend to respond best to people much like themselves. Poor people and old people have quality medical care available to them, but they sometimes do not get it. Often, they are patronized. Said one doctor, "what you have to realize is that poor people are often *poor* people." On the other hand, some don't get care because they don't know how to seek it. Institutions dealing with the old and the poor can do a real service by informing their clients of their rights and privileges and how to get them.

Most of our respondents reported that they took care of patients even if they could not pay, and half thought their patients were aware of this. Actually 80 percent of patients believe this of their own doctors. They were confident that if they could not pay their bills, their doctor would work something out for them. But only 50 percent believed it of doctors in general. Nearly 50 percent of the doctors admitted they didn't comply with Medicare regulations, and two-thirds thought patients would understand how difficult it was to follow federal regulations and excuse them for not complying. Only one-fourth of the patients believed this about their own doctors, but more than 40 percent indicted doctors in general.

One-third of the doctors reported they do not like to treat old people. For one thing, respondents reported, old people tend to be cranky and unpleasant and have a tendency to die of their ailments. Furthermore, a great many old people are also poor.

The problem of treatment of women has been the object of considerable concern. Many women's magazines have run articles alleging women are treated poorly by physicians. Nearly half of the doctors admit they treat men better than women but only one-third believe patients would hold them culpable. Both the male and female doctors we interviewed seemed to agree that woman patients tended to be more querulous, complaining, and emotional than men.

There is little doubt that doctors prefer to deal with people with whom they feel compatible. We did not include special groups in our research because we were trying to discover "mainstream" issues. There was enough irritation expressed by both doctors and patients to suggest that the old, the poor, and the female often experience interpersonal "events" that interfere with good medical care. It may be that these groups find it difficult, if not impossible, to develop working relationships with their physicians. Clearly there are prejudices that demand investigation and repair.

Ambience. Courtesy and office management are important issues in doctor-patient relationships. For example, most patients believed that doctors were not considerate of their time. Doctors unanimously expressed concern with the amount of time they gave to each patient. They justified brief encounters by pointing to their patient load. Only 40 percent of the patients believed their own doctors give them enough time and most charged doctors, specialists particularly, with being inconsiderate with time. Long waits and short visits seem to be the norm reported. It is not clear, though, how much time doctors actually do give. The issue may be one of perceptions. Doctors feel pressured to move on to the next case, patients feel urgent about getting more information and consolation. Thus neither side can be satisfied.

MELISSA K. (ELEMENTARY TEACHER), AGED THIRTY-TWO

When I went to my doctor because there was blood in my urine he seemed very concerned. He examined me and then he suggested that I see a urologist. He had his secretary call and get me an appointment, and I got in to see the urologist the next day, but I had to go at 7:30 in the morning because that was when the urologist took initial referrals from other doctors. The urologist sent me off to the hospital lab for tests and told me to call for an appointment so he could interpret the tests. I did what he told me, but when I called for an appointment I was told he would be out of town for a week and no one could report on the test results until he came back. I didn't think to call my own doctor. I waited for him and the pain got worse. I finally called my own doctor who got access to the tests and told me what was wrong and suggested that I wait it out. However uncomfortable it was, he told me, it wasn't disastrous. So I waited and worried and then one morning I passed a kidney stone and then I felt better. When I finally got to see the urologist he told me that I should probably pass a kidney stone soon. I told him I already did and he asked me why I took his time with the appointment, then, when other people were urgent to see him.

Some specialists define their job as interpretation of test and examination results and nothing more. They literally treat organs, not patients. While considerable work with specialists on interpersonal relationships might be profitable, the most obvious answer for patients is to rely on their personal doctor as an information filter and support. Most internists and family physicians define this as a major role they play on behalf of their patients.

Hospital care is another source of irritation. Most patients do not understand what their doctor is doing for them when they are in the hospital. Many are resentful of the charges made for hospital visits. Doctors reported they were compelled to move rapidly on their hospital rounds and felt pressured by the process.

WILLIAM P. (INTERNAL MEDICINE), AGED FORTY-SIX

You want to know how I use my time at the hospital. Well, here it is. Each day of the week I make hospital rounds at 7:30

A.M. *and see every patient I have in the hospital. For each pa-*
tient, first, I look at the chart to find out what happened last
night. Reading the nurses notes is frequently the only way to
find out what really happened. Then, it's off to see the patient
and ask him how he was the previous evening. Sometimes it is
necessary to do all or part of a physical to check on progress or
problems. Then, I return to the nurses station, write a note in
the chart, write orders so the nurses will know what to do
next, check all the laboratory values, and then repeat the whole
procedure with the next patient. If I have to call a relative or
contact social services to arrange for special care on discharge,
then much more time must be allowed to make "rounds" on
that patient. I know that all the patient sees is a brief visit,
sometimes no more than once a day, and I know it leads to a
great deal of discontent because the patient would like to have
me at his side, but there doesn't seem to be any way to let the
patient know how much time in-hospital care really takes if
done properly. This doesn't even include the time required to
dictate an admission summary and a discharge summary. If
only my patients knew the untold hours spent out of their sight
making sure all is well, they would be more satisfied with my
services.

Physicians could do a considerably better job of explanation on
this count, and hospitals could help by providing patients with
pamphlets explaining what goes on behind the scenes on their
behalf while they are in the hospital.

Problems in Social Status

Most doctors are aware of their status and depend on it to help
them impress their patients. However, status differences can interfere with effective communication. Many patients find it hard
to talk to their doctors, especially to ask questions. They feel their
doctors talk down to them, patronize them, and confuse them
with technical talk.

Three-fourths of the doctors surveyed believed they were more
intelligent than their patients and nearly 100 percent of the doctors
expect their patients to believe this. Sixty percent of the patients

agreed, although some hedged, saying doctors were better trained in a specialized area. We found a sizable vocal minority who were very hostile to doctors because of "their superior attitude." Most of those did not have regular doctors.

The main problem presented by status differences is the effect it has on information exchange. A patient can withhold information if he believes the doctor does not take him seriously. Most patients reported they do not feel completely free to talk about their problems. They offer remarks like, "I never know whether what I say makes sense" or "I get the idea he is impatient while I am talking." Many rely on their doctors' questions and do not offer information unless it is asked for. Patients tend not to ask questions, and if given the opportunity to talk freely, they are likely to express their feelings about their illness rather than inform the doctor about the details. This can have serious ramifications, for the doctor can only work with the information he has. Training physicians in sophisticated techniques of history taking might do a great deal to bridge the status gap between them and their patients.

Nearly all of our physician respondents reported their social contacts are mostly with other physicians, and more than half rejected all social contact with their patients. Furthermore, they expected their patients to respect this social distance. Seventy percent of the doctors expected their patients to avoid direct contact should they encounter each other in social situations. Many reported they will give no more than a nod of acknowledgment. Doctors are also defensive about talking medicine with patients outside the office. Some report they are concerned about possible malpractice actions if they make professional comments inappropriately. Others believe people take advantage of them at social gatherings and try to milk them for free advice.

Three-fourths of the patients reported their own doctors maintain this social detachment and nearly all patients resented the doctors' social separateness. Many doctors felt victimized because their patients saw them as stereotypes. Some felt pressured to live up to their media image. But they may have overestimated the hostility directed at them. The pervasive finding through our studies was that patients who had an opportunity to build a relationship with a doctor were satisfied with it. Less than 25 percent expressed lack of confidence in their own doctor. More important, less than one-third were willing to express lack of confidence in the medical professional in general. Patients understand that doctors are a special class with special knowledge.

Problems in Financing Medical Care

Money is a major obstacle to doctor-and-patient collaboration. In general, patients are not particularly sympathetic to the economic pressures their doctors claim, and many potential patients reject medical care because they feel they cannot afford it. Sometimes doctors recommend expensive treatments and tests without considering the burden their recommendations place on their patients. Finally, many patients are confused about their medical insurance plans and avoid necessary medical care because they cannot manage the claim forms.

Nearly 80 percent of the doctors reported they believed patients thought fees were too high. They defended their fees on the grounds that their education was expensive, their cost of operation high, and their services valuable. Patients in our surveys seemed unable to swallow these arguments, despite the fact they were covered by insurance. Two-thirds of our respondents complained about their own physicians charges. They were unanimous that medical care costs too much. Furthermore, though they agreed that medical care was valuable, they resented what appeared to them to be doctors taking advantage of their sickness. It appeared that when patients are sick they pay the fee to get the service they need, but when they feel well they are very concerned about the high cost of medical care. Three-fourths of the doctors reported that their patients generally found it hard to pay the fees, even those covered by insurance. Almost 100 percent of the patients believe that doctors are the highest paid occupational group and they resented the fact that doctors got their money from the misery of others.

A great many people have much of their medical costs covered by insurance, but as we surveyed our patient population we found more than half of them did not know what their medical plans covered nor did they know how to make claims. A good program educating patients on how to use their medical insurance would probably do a lot to improve relationships between doctors and at least some of their patients.

Problems Arising from Ethical Issues

The practice of medicine is a life-and-death occupation. In a typical intensive care facility of a large hospital, there are several rooms each containing a human being, usually completely immobilized, with tubes coming out of every aperture, needles in veins, breathing apparatuses, oxygen masks, and monitors of various sorts. The humans look like cyborgs, part person, part machine. They are being kept alive while physicians do their work. Surgeons repair broken parts, specialists of various sorts provide treatments, the whole operation integrated so that a life is saved. The current wave of artificial heart "installations" keep people alive via connection to a mechanical device. Kidney dialysis is an even more common form of human-machine integration.

Doctors are concerned with both the technical issue of how to sustain life and the moral issue of its quality, should it be sustained. Whether or not to use life-support systems and when to turn them off represent formidable life-and-death confrontations. The ailments of the ordinary patient seem trivial to the doctor preoccupied with a patient hovering on the edge of death. Patients do not seem to have a sense that they might, someday, confront such major decisions themselves. It is one thing to talk about these issues abstractly, something else again when we must face them. The problem is, doctors face such issues all the time though patients face them only once.

Virtually all doctors and patients believed in the principle of confidentiality. There was considerable disagreement and misunderstanding on what that means. The most important misunderstanding was from patients who believed they were *not* entitled to information about their own case. Doctors, on one hand, are quite clear that no one should have access to patient records without patient permission. It is customary, for example, when a specialist is called into a case, for the patient to give approval for the transfer or sharing of records.

The issue of what patients are entitled to know versus what is it good for them to know divided our respondents. Most doctors claimed they told the whole truth to their patients. Several reported they were often very careful about what they said and how they said it, however. Many believed they had some patients who could not tolerate full disclosure about their medical conditions. For those patients, doctors filtered information, giving out only what was necessary to explain treatments. A few, however, were quite blunt about the way they gave information.

ALMA H. (SECRETARY), AGED FIFTY-FIVE

I found out about my lung cancer on a Tuesday morning when Dr. D. called and said, "Alma, you flunked your chest X ray." I had just had a routine physical. The news was like a bomb. I didn't feel sick. Dr. D. had been after me for a couple of years to give up smoking. The next thing he said was, "see, I told you those cigarettes were going to get you." It was cruel. That is no way to get a death sentence.

Relationships with family represent another serious ethical issue. While doctors are generally very careful about holding patient information confidential in all cases, a few feel patients' families should be informed and involved in case management. Sometimes the patient doesn't want the family to know. It is very hard to decide how much information should be given to whom and in what way. A few doctors indicated they discussed the matter of information with their patients, but this was a very small minority. They all noted that it took a great deal of time to handle information this way and that they often made mistakes in deciding whom to trust.

Second opinions. There was more disagreement about second opinions than we expected. Half of our medical respondents found second opinions a nuisance.

DR. HAROLD V. (SURGEON), AGED FORTY-EIGHT

Let's face it. I tell a person he needs to have his gall bladder snipped out. So he says, "I want a second opinion." So I say,

OK, you need more vitamins. "Ha, ha," he says, "but seriously, Doc, don't I need a second opinion to think this out." What kind of second opinion? I send him to a friend of mine for a second opinion, so to do it right, the friend has to do all the tests and examinations and sock the man with a big bill. So he calls me and says, let me see the patient's records. So I show him the records. Do you think he is going to question my diagnosis? So the patient goes out of town to somebody in another city who doesn't know him at all. Once again, he pays for the whole medical work-up. So the guy either confirms my diagnosis or he tries to talk the man out of it. He maybe says, it can be handled medically. So now my patient is in trouble. What does he do? Is he going to go to the guy in the other city who thinks it could be managed medically. He comes back to me and tells me and I stick to my guns. I'm a surgeon. When a gall bladder is that bad, it comes out. Where is the patient going to go? Second opinion sounds easy but it is not as simple as you think it is.

Patients are also divided about the matter. Nearly half responded that they were prepared to accept their own doctor's recommendation without question. Second opinion meant that they were to be inconvenienced by the time and expense of another medical examination when the second doctor would merely ratify their own doctor's recommendations. Furthermore, most patients reported they would not know how to handle it, if the two doctors disagreed. Finally, a strong minority, nearly 40 percent, believed that second opinions represented a form of fee-splitting, a way to get more money into medical circulation.

Suspicions of collusion. More than 50 percent of the patients surveyed believed doctors cover up for each other. Patients tended to believe that malpractice suits were justified because they tended to crack the wall of defense that physicians put up about the quality of medical practice. Patients are generally unaware of quality controls imposed on physicians and most do not know what to do if they have a complaint. Thus the legal profession presents a real alternative to a patient who believes he or she has been badly treated.

Doctors are acutely aware of the issue. More than half believed that they do cover up for one another. Some sample quotes are indicative. "Patients are really not qualified to evaluate our work." "We have to protect the right to make a mistake, otherwise we'd be sued out of existence." "I don't dare criticize someone else's work. They would get me back." Furthermore, nearly 90 percent of the doctors surveyed suspected that patients believed they covered up for one another.

The question of evaluation of physician performance represents the most pervasive ethical issue in the practice of medicine. Patients do not know their rights. Physicians do not know whom to trust. And, the society is litigious. There may be special cases of total trust between doctors and patients, but the patterns of responses we received from patients seemed to indicate that they would *like to trust* their physicians, not that they did. Doctors, on the other hand, generally felt hampered in their activity by the possibility that their patients might take extreme action in the event of perception of error.

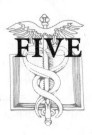

FIVE

Obtaining Quality Medical Care

In the previous chapter, we specified two criteria for a good medical relationship. First, your doctor must be competent. Second, you and your doctor must be able to work out a genuine collaboration on your behalf. In chapter 3 we explained how to identify a competent physician. This chapter explains what you can do to help your doctor provide you with the best of care.

Selecting a Doctor

The most important finding in our study of doctors and patients was that the best medical care results from a long-term relationship between doctor and patient. People with no regular doctor or those who jump from doctor to doctor have more complaints about their medical care than those who sustain a relationship with one doctor over a long period of time. You cannot pick your doctor at random out of a phone book. Selection of a doctor requires expenditure of both time and money.

Because you share your doctor's time with many other patients, you must be sure he will give you a fair share of time and attention. It is most efficient to pick a good doctor on the first try, but it is not advisable to wait until you have a medical problem. You may not get the best choice, or any choice, on the spur of the moment. Hospital emergency rooms generally respond well to the unexpected, but the doctors there do not offer long-term care. To ensure that you will not have to rely on a stranger at a crucial moment, establish, as soon as possible, a relationship with a competent doctor in whom you have confidence.

The most valuable service a personal doctor can provide is knowledge of the continuity of your health and sickness. When you are seriously ill and you go to a doctor who does not know you, it is impossible for him to take the kind of complete medical history that facilitates effective diagnosis and treatment. He must work with what he can learn quickly and often must rely on your brief report and laboratory tests to make a diagnosis. He may not understand the subtleties of your physiology as only your personal doctor can. The emergency doctor literally patches you up as best he can and passes you on to another doctor or back to your regular doctor. An emergency room is valuable when you are away from home and your usual medical support system is not available, but it is not a substitute for regular medical care.

Your personal physician is not only the first line of treatment for your illness but also the coordinator of your care should you suffer a serious illness. She can diagnose and treat most of your illnesses, refer you to specialists, stand by during surgery, supervise your stay in the hospital, interpret your condition to your family or loved ones, and provide you with thorough and systematic explanations of your condition, your treatment, and the possible outcome of your case. The relationship develops gradually. When you are relatively young, you may only see your doctor for an occasional flu or sprained ankle. Even these sporadic encounters will enable her to learn something about you and your personality, and you to learn something about how she practices medicine. As you grow older and acquire illnesses, a doctor who is familiar with you and your medical history can respond in a fully informed manner.

DR. KENDALL T. (GENERAL PRACTICE), AGED SEVENTY

The thing I regretted most about retiring was what happened to some of the patients I have been following for years.

*There are a number of families where I was treating three gen-
erations. The grandparents came to me as newlyweds, and now
I was treating their grandchildren. I think I practiced very good
medicine with these people because I understood them. I did
not have to struggle to find things out. I had it all in my records and I knew how to use it. For their part, they knew how
they could reach me. I could do a lot over the phone and not
charge them for it. I knew everything about Billy Decker's
liver, and I knew exactly when to worry about Edna Kline's
kidneys. I really didn't have too many emergency decisions to
make, I could head things off before they happened. That is the
best kind of medicine. I am really impressed by some of these
schools that are training specialists in family medicine, because
it proves to me that my career was not wasted. I still think the
kind of medicine where you know your patients in detail is the
best kind of medicine.*

Like Dr. T. your personal doctor will take your peculiarities
and special problems into account. The number of contacts you
have with your doctor will increase as you grow older. Your doctor
will accumulate information on your life-style, the way you respond to medications, and your preferences in treatment that can
improve your care as you acquire chronic illnesses. Furthermore,
your relationship will enable him to instruct you and even "nag"
you a little about smoking, drinking, the way your eat, or anything
you are doing that might impair your health.

Your personal physician can also develop contact with your
family. If you are ever so sick that decisions must be made by
someone else, the fact that your doctor knows your family im-
proves the chances that decisions about your treatment can be
made that suit your preferences. You can also share your private
thoughts about what you want to have happen in the event of
catastrophic illness and, to some extent, how you wish your death
to be handled. If you have a living will, your doctor can help
execute it.

Three circumstances may arise where you have no choice in
doctors. First, in any emergency service, whether hospital or free-
standing, you will be assigned to whichever doctor is available.
Second, if you belong to a prepaid plan, you may be assigned to

a doctor. Third, if you live where there are very few doctors, your choice is restricted to the doctors in the vicinity. In these circumstances it is particularly important that you be prepared to provide information and ask questions.

Ask your friends. The choice of a doctor is in your hands. You can get information and advice from others, but it is the information you get from professional contact that is most important to your decision. People talk a lot about their illnesses and their doctors. Several of our respondents told us that as they got older they found themselves discussing their symptoms and medical experiences with their friends. One respondent referred to these conversations as "organ recitals." If you listen to these conversations carefully, you can get some useful information. On the other hand, bear in mind that people tend to be defensive about their doctors, as they are about the gas mileage their cars get or how their children are doing in school.

You are most likely to hear stories of miracles or horrors. Accounts of routine good care and uneventful healing do not make good party talk. You may hear one person report being insulted by a doctor, while another will talk about exceptional sensitivity the same doctor showed. It's helpful to keep in mind that whatever happens between doctor and patient usually has something to do with the mix of their personalities. In any given case, it could be different for you. On the other hand, if you hear one doctor consistently praised another condemned, you have some useful information.

Check standard references. A great many medical sources advise you to select a doctor based on recommendation of the local medical society. However, the medical society will tell you nothing about quality. They will give you names, addresses, and specialties, essentially the same information you can get from the yellow pages of the phone directory. The most important information you can get from the phone book is location. If convenient access is important to you, the phone book can provide a starting list of physicians with the proper specialty and convenient locations.

Medical societies will also provide information about degrees, residencies, and licensing. If you suspect a doctor's background, you can usually get accurate information about it from the medical society. The information you get from the medical society does not guarantee selection of a competent doctor but can provide basic information about competency. The phone book tells you only name, address, and medical specialty. If location is a concern, however, you can confine your further investigations to doctors whose offices you can reach easily.

It is important to select a doctor with the appropriate kind of practice for your needs. In most cases, an internist or general practitioner is best. It is not advisable to select a specialist unless you have a disease that requires constant management and your specialist is also willing to deal with your other medical concerns. Some chronic diseases, arthritis and diabetes, for example, can provide the focus for general treatment by a specialist.

If you have children, a family practitioner can coordinate medical care for every member of the family. You may prefer to have a pediatrician for the children and an internist for yourself. Both pediatricians and internists practice general medicine but restrict their practice by age group (internists specialize in adults; pediatricians in children).

Questions to ask. Once you have a list of doctors from which to choose, check carefully for anything that might disqualify or recommend them. If you can get a personal reference from a friend or acquaintance, ask specific questions. How does your friend use the doctor? Occasionally for acute illness? For a chronic condition? What has the doctor done and how satisfied has your friend been with it? Don't be satisfied simply with a song of praise. Ask what kind of relationship he or she has with the doctor. What do they talk about during an office visit? What does the doctor do during an examination? How much time is spent with you? Check on what the doctor has recommended, how it worked, and how the doctor follows up. Next, have your friend describe precisely what goes on when he calls for an appointment. How easy is it to reach the doctor? How long do you have to wait for an appointment? How promptly does the doctor keep the appointments? Ask, also, about the fee and how it is paid. Does the doctor bill patients? Take credit cards? Ask for payment at each visit?

Evaluate the responses on your own criteria. For example, none of the payment alternatives are necessarily good or bad, but you may have your own preferences about paying, and as long as you have a choice, you can select a doctor that suits your method of financial management. Keep track of the answers you get to your questions and, if and when you encounter the doctor, compare your experiences with the reports you received.

Be somewhat cautious, however, about friends' reports. People have a natural tendency to try to confirm their own beliefs by talking other people into them. If someone lacks confidence in his doctor, he can compensate for it and reassure himself by talking you into choosing him. It is often useful to ask your friend directly, "would you take responsibility for recommending that I go to this doctor?" If your friend has any unexpressed doubts, they will emerge in the answer to this question.

Exploratory contact. Even if you have personal references, it is a good idea to make a trial appointment to check out the doctors on your list firsthand. Check first to make sure that the doctor is taking new patients. If she is, get what information you can over the phone. The receptionist can provide a great deal of information about how the doctor carries on her practice. Ask her how long you would have to wait for a regular appointment and how long she spends with the average patient. Request information about fee structure, hospital affiliations, and coverage when the doctor is off. If the information sounds satisfactory, make an appointment, but make sure the receptionist knows that the visit is exploratory. Simply explain that you are looking for a personal physician and you would like to come in for a visit so you can discuss possibilities. You may have to make trial visits to three or four physicians before you are ready to make a choice. The visits may not be covered by your insurance plan, but the expense is well worth it, if it helps you choose wisely.

A few doctors have prospective new patients come in for an orientation visit, for which they rarely charge. During this visit, the doctor inquires about why you are seeking a doctor and the policies and procedures of his practice. If you are fortunate enough to find a doctor who operates this way, you can get firsthand information about qualifications and personality by spending a little time together.

The first thing to find out at the initial visit is how you feel about the physician as a human being. Listen to the way he talks, to the kinds of questions he asks, how he makes you feel. Ask yourself if you would feel comfortable telling this person some of your most intimate secrets. If you are not satisfied at the very beginning, chances are you will find fault with his work later. In special cases, a physician may be so competent with your particular problem that personality ceases to be an issue.

Base your decision on your own preferences. Some people work best with physicians who are matter-of-fact or authoritarian. Others prefer those who are relatively nondirective. Some choose doctors who provide a great deal of information or permit you to ask questions freely. Make sure you know what you are looking for in a doctor, given that you can't have Marcus Welby.

The second thing to find out is whether the doctor's professional policies suit your preferences. Ask about important issues such as how appointments are made, how long you have to wait until you get one, what happens when you get there, how long you will wait in the waiting room, how much time you will normally have with the physician, and what the procedures are for getting information, asking questions, and sustaining contact.

You should be able to get an appointment immediately, if you are very sick. Most doctors have a set of priorities for urgent cases. At most, you should be able to see your doctor within three days. You should not have to wait more than an hour at the time of an appointment. Actually, the average is thirty minutes, but sometimes there are emergencies that throw the schedule off. You should expect fifteen to twenty minutes of actual contact time. It is also important to inquire about phone contact. The effective practice of medicine requires that you be able to get your questions answered promptly and that you provide relevant information to the doctor regularly.

You will also want to know about hospital affiliations, what other doctors she is associated with, who handles calls when she is off, and how emergencies are handled. You should come away assured that if you appear in the hospital emergency room, your doctor will be notified and take over the case. You should also know precisely whom to call, if your doctor is off. If you cannot get answers to these questions, it is probably risky to select that doctor.

Third, make sure you understand the fee structure and can accommodate it. Doctors charge according to time and expertise. Fees are usually consistent within economic market areas. Most distinguish between a short, intermediate, and long visit. You should be able to get a definition of what the doctor does during each type of visit and check with other doctors to make sure the fees are consistent with standard practice in the area. Short visits for blood pressure checks, shots, etc., are often gratis or cost only for the materials used. Be suspicious if the doctor does not discriminate between short and intermediate visits. Costs can mount rapidly if you need regular care and must pay full price for short visits.

Inquire about the cost of a complete examination and what it includes. Some physicians conduct an extended evaluation when accepting new patients. This is often expensive, but once the initial evaluation is complete, annual examinations are not required. It is a good idea to check the fee schedule for hospital visits and special tests and analyses. Inquire about what laboratories and X ray services the doctor uses and what their charges are.

You will also need information about method of payment. Some doctors expect payment when service is rendered. They will give you receipts indicating the services they perform and the cost and expect you to fill out insurance forms for your reimbursement. Some will fill out the forms and submit them for their reimbursement, and if they are not reimbursed in full, they will bill you for the difference. Some will accept "assignment," that is, take whatever the insurance company or Medicare pays for the service. Others will bill you for the difference.

You should also know what the doctor's policy is if exceptional circumstances should arise and you are unable to pay for care at the time it is given.

Fourth, establish at the initial visit that the doctor regards your expectations as reasonable. Tell your doctor what you expect from him. Some doctors may not be prepared to give you the kind of treatment you want. By asking, you can find out whether your expectations are reasonable. If none of the doctors on your list are prepared to meet your criteria, you might have to reexamine what you expect. You should also ask what he expects from you. By sharing information about goals, you can discover if a mutual commitment is possible.

Once you have decided on a doctor, make an initial appointment. In most cases, this involves a complete history and physical examination, which serve as a base line for your subsequent treatment. Use your first appointment to establish the rules of the relationship. From your first interview and your first visit, you should have the answers to the following questions.

1. What do you need to know about me that you do not already know? Be ready to provide your doctor with the information he requests.
2. What are your rules for calling you? When do you want me to call? What information should I have ready when I call?
3. Who takes your place when you are off duty, out of town, or on vacation? What information does he or she have about me? Can I get to you if it is a real emergency?
4. What role do you want members of my family to play in my medical care? (If you have instructions about who is to know and do what, be sure to write them out and give them to your doctor. If you have special instructions about organ donations or heroic measures if your life is in danger, be sure to write out a living will and make sure your doctor will honor it.)
5. Do I have quirks that make it difficult for you to treat me? What are they?
6. What would you like me to learn in order to become a better patient?
7. I have some comments about the way you and your office operate. Are you willing to listen to me?

You may think of more questions. Be sure you understand the answers you are given. Take written notes on what your doctor tells you. As an informed user of medical care, you can exert considerable control over the nature of the agreement between you and your doctor. Use it to build your medical safety net so you have confidence that if you become ill, you have competent service available.

Preparing for Your Visits

Making an appointment with a physician is not a casual act. You seek an appointment because something is wrong. It is important that your doctor knows precisely what is bothering you. It helps to prepare in advance.

The rhetoric of medical care. Effective interpersonal communication is based on the ancient Greek art of "rhetoric," defined as "the art of finding in any given case, all the available means of persuasion." Effective interpersonal communication with your doctor means that you know how to explain what you want from him and know how to respond to facilitate his providing it. This means you must have reasonable expectations and understand the constraints of the situation. Bluntly speaking, you must be prepared to make maximum use of the limited time you have.

There are five basic features of every doctor-patient relationship. First, it virtually always happens in the doctor's facilities (the office, the emergency room, the hospital). Second, Doctors do not solicit patients; they wait for you to come to them. Third, you must share your doctor's time with a great many other people. Fourth, there are limits on what your doctor can do for you. Fifth, your doctor depends on you for all basic information about your case.

The first step in preparation is to define your complaint. Your doctor will respond to what he thinks is important in what you say. You must be direct and to the point. If you mince words, use euphemisms, or conceal information, you can mislead your doctor into a defective diagnosis. The bottom line is to get the facts straight.

WINIFRED J., M.D. (INTERNAL MEDICINE), AGED FORTY

I saw an article in a popular magazine that told about a patient who came to the doctor with a mole that was worrying him. He was under treatment for arthritis and when he came in he talked about his arthritis. According to the article, the doc-

tor questioned him about his arthritis but never asked about the mole. I wondered how the doctor could ask about the mole, if he never knew the patient had a mole that worried him. People are constantly charging us with overlooking important symptoms, but we cannot take a symptom into account unless the patient calls it to our attention. All we can do is ask the patient to tell us what's wrong. We have no choice but to depend on the answer. We cannot see through clothing and we cannot read minds.

Planned talk is the most effective way to accomplish interpersonal goals. Both parties can contribute to the success or failure of a medical visit. If you can focus your doctor's attention on your real problem, you raise the chances of a satisfactory outcome. Wrong cues might result in unnecessary investigation, expensive testing, and ineffective treatment.

It helps if your personality meshes with your doctor's.

HARRIS P. (ENGINEER), AGED FIFTY

I liked Dr. Y. He was tough and brusque. He didn't beat around the bush. He would open with "what's wrong," and I'd tell him and he'd have a couple of ideas of what to do about it. He'd give the pros and cons and then I'd be out of there. I liked the fact that he had respect for my intelligence.

GLENDA P. (COMPUTER PROGRAMMER), AGED FORTY-SEVEN

I went to Dr. Y because my husband liked him so much. I had these headaches once and I tripped a few times, and I thought they had something to do with my new eyeglasses but he demanded that I have some X rays of my head, and he just wouldn't let me talk about the problem. He was too quick to jump to conclusions and he treated me like a fool.

Dr. Y. used a pattern of interaction that he found generally effective. He did not realize that some patients did not fit his stereotypes. Though some of his patients liked the way he handled himself, Glenda P. did not. If you were Glenda P., could you persuade Dr. Y. to meet your needs? Would you even try?

Communication goals must be set within a range of the possible. Every doctor-patient relationship occurs in short, well-defined episodes. They open with the question about your condition and end with a recommendation. If important information is concealed, the transaction fails. Your doctor will expect you to present a complaint. He will listen for you to say something like, "I hurt," "I feel sick," "I am unhappy." He will then ask some questions, perhaps examine you, and make recommendations. You and he both presume that you will improve as a result of following the advice.

The situation can be more complicated. You may be sicker than you or the doctor expected, or your doctor may require more information to make a diagnosis. If you need tests or even hospitalization, he will ask for your authorization, and if you give it (in writing), he will take charge. You may feel pressured and rushed. At this point, your ability to ask questions is very important.

Your desire for a quick cure may lead you to overestimate what your doctor can do for you. It may frustrate you if your doctor announces, "time will make it go away; just rest and drink liquids." You may believe this is not enough help or consolation. You believe your doctor can do more. "Why," you ask yourself, "is he withholding treatment from me? What does he have against me?" Sulking won't help, but a realistic outlook might.

DR. ANNETTE F. (GENERAL PRACTICE), AGED THIRTY-FIVE

My patients sometimes go to great lengths to get me to prescribe something for them. When I won't write a prescription, they will sometimes ask, "should I buy nose drops or cough syrup at the drugstore?" I say, "no," and they ask, "well can I take aspirin?" I say, "it probably won't hurt you, if you are in pain, but it won't cure you. You have a cold and it will go away." I sometimes run down a list of things for the patient to keep track of. "Do you cough up colored mucous." "Are you running a fever?" "Do you have chest pain?" But some of my patients will tell me what they think I want to hear even when it isn't true. I find it hard to get some patients home without writing them a prescription of some sort.

Doctors can do only do what they are trained to do: diagnose, advise, and follow up. They can discuss your problem, define it, and offer recommendations. Doctors may differ in the manner in which they do this, but however they do it, the process of diagnosis and treatment largely depends on *you*. You decide how to answer the questions, whether to take the pills, go to the lab, enter the hospital, or have the surgery. You can ask questions and discuss major disagreements, or you can leave the office and never return.

If you choose to accept the advice, keep your doctor posted. If the treatment works, your report helps your doctor know what to do the next time the problem arises. If it does not, your report suggests an alternative. It is especially important to notify your doctor, if the treatment causes problems. The best treatment does the job with minimal side effects.

The form on page 143 is provided as a guide in preparing for visits to your doctor. Make copies and fill one out before each visit to the doctor. Put a copy with your medical records. Your doctor may want to keep the one you bring to add to your medical history file. If you are not feeling well enough to fill out this form yourself, ask for help. If you can, take notes on what your doctor tells for your own guidance and to keep your records complete.

Fill out this form for each visit. Take your time and fill it out carefully. It is sometimes difficult to describe how you feel subjectively. People experience pain and discomfort in very different ways. The form is designed to help you detail your complaint. If you fill it out carefully, it will help you define what to say when you see the doctor. Keep it with you when you go, as a reminder, so you do not leave out any important information.

Making contact. The person who answers the phone at your doctor's office understands your doctor's appointment system. A typical priority list might include instructions to schedule seriously ill patients in the morning and follow-ups in the afternoon. Calls from the hospital about critical patients are usually put through immediately. Calls with reports or questions about treatment are noted, and the doctor calls back at intervals.

You get the best service from the receptionist if you understand the rules. In any case, make your requests simple and don't get

THIS IS MY PROBLEM

State the problem. _____
When did it start? _____
Do you feel pain? _____ Where? _____
Can you point to it? _____ What kind of pain is it? Sharp, piercing,
dull, throbbing? _____ Steady or intermittent? _____
Shooting? _____ Describe its pattern _____
When do you feel it? When you exercise? After meals? When you are
lying down? All the time? Other (Describe in detail) _____
Fill in details similar to the above for each of the following possibilities
that might be relevant in your case.
Nausea _____
Vomiting _____
Fatigue _____
Sleep problems _____
General feeling of uneasiness or anxiety _____
Depression _____
Diarrhea _____
Constipation _____
Itching, rash _____
Feeling faint _____
Vision problem _____
Hearing problem _____
Sneezing, coughing, wheezing _____
Other (Describe in detail) _____
Was there some event that set it off? _____
Did it come on suddenly or gradually? _____
Has it gotten worse? _____

Did you ever have it before? _____
When and under what circumstances? _____
How does it hamper you? _____
Did you ever see a doctor about it? _____ Who and when? _____
What was the diagnosis? _____
What did the doctor tell you to do about it? _____
Did you do it? _____ What was the result? _____
Are you taking any over-the-counter drugs for it? _____
With what results? _____
List all the drugs you are currently taking and bring them to the visit.

List all the drugs to which you are allergic. _____
List all medical conditions for which you are currently being treated.

irritated if you are asked for information. The receptionist gets her instructions about what to say and what to ask from the doctor. There is no point in resenting her.

Get a sense of when your doctor returns phone calls. Most of them do it on a regular schedule. When you call for information, ask the receptionist when the doctor is likely to call back, then try to be around for the call. If your call is not returned promptly, call back.

CANDACE W. (SECRETARY-RECEPTIONIST), AGED SIXTY-TWO

Some patients are just awful. They patronize me, yell at me, and sometimes act like I don't exist. When they think the bill is too high they yell at me. When the doctor doesn't call them back right away they call over and over and blame me for not giving him the message. Many will not even learn my name. Some patients are so nice, I may slip their notes to the top of the pile. I don't treat the others unfairly, but I certainly won't do anything special for them.

There is no need for reticence about discussing your needs with the receptionist or secretary. They are trained to respond to emergencies and usually can manage the doctor's time. When you call, keep your visit preparation form in front of you, so you can supply information quickly and accurately. Simply report your symptoms. Providing your own diagnosis, such as, "I've had this cold for a week and I think I ought to be looked at," may get you a deferred appointment, since you have already identified a nonemergent condition. "I have had a painful sore throat and fever for two days" may get you rapid treatment because of the indication of a more urgent condition. "I've just been feeling miserable lately" may evoke immediate concern from some receptionists, but it helps if you explain how urgent you feel about your condition. Be cautious about calling something an emergency. If you erroneously claim an emergency too many times, it may be hard to get the staff to take you seriously when the real thing happens.

As you gain experience with your doctor's staff, you will learn what information to give them when you call for an appointment, as well as how much consideration they will give to your personal or work concerns when they schedule you. You will also get a sense of what your doctor regards as worthy of an immediate appointment, and what can wait a day or two.

Keep courtesy in mind in dealing with your doctor's staff. They frequently get a hard time from callers. A major university runs a series of workshops for people who work for doctors. They are called "flack-catchers' workshops" and are designed to teach medical-support personnel how to handle the anger and frustration vented on them by patients unhappy because they waited too long for, or had an unsatisfactory encounter with, the doctor. The doctor's staff can help you get quality service from your doctor. But they do not set policies; they cannot violate the rules of their job on your behalf. Furthermore, if you take out your anger on them you can materially interfere with your chances of getting service the next time. If you are angry with your doctor you must deal directly with your doctor. It does not help to push around or verbally abuse receptionists and nurses.

Each medical office runs differently, but the one fact you can be sure of is that "waiting rooms" are properly named. Doctors are rarely on time for their appointments. It is not that they plan to be late. Most of the time they cannot predict how long they will spend with a given case. Most allot a specific amount of time to each patient based on the complaint, and then try to build cushions into the day so they can catch up with themselves. But if a complicated case presents itself or if an extra appointment has to be scheduled, everyone has to wait. Rarely do miracles happen and the day runs on time. This means you have to be on time for appointments, whether or not the doctor is.

In addition, do not rely on the doctor's supply of magazines or books to amuse you. Because you know you are going to have to spend a little waiting time, be sure to bring along something you enjoy doing to help you spend the time. Above all, do not allow anxiety and irritation to rise to a point where it interferes with information exchange. Being angry, as well as sick, when you get to see the doctor diminishes your return on the time allotted.

Facilitating Diagnosis and Treatment

SOAP stands for Subjective Objective Assessment Plan. Many doctors base their investigation and diagnosis on this system. *Subjective* refers to the history and description presented by the patient. *Objective* consists of the various examinations, measurements, observations, and tests made by the physician during the examination. *Assessment* refers to the diagnosis. *Plan* is the recommended treatment.

Your medical history. We have pointed out several times how important the medical history is. It is important to give your doctor all the help you can during history taking. You can do this best by being prepared.

It is important that your personal doctor have a complete and accurate history. You should have a copy in case you ever have to change doctors. Remember, you have a right to your records, and you must take them with you or make them available when you see a doctor other than your own. Gather and keep your medical history in a file at home. If you need a consultation with a specialist or are hospitalized, someone should know where your records are so they can be provided promptly. As the years pass, your home copy should grow with each medical encounter. Keep records along with your doctor. If your doctor should retire or move, make sure you get your records so they can be easily transferred to your next doctor. Legally, ownership of medical records resides with the writer, e.g., hospital, laboratory, or doctor, but you are legally entitled to a copy of any record pertaining to you.

Doctors have reported that many patients, for one reason or another, conceal important information. Your doctor must know of all your past illnesses, even the embarrassing ones. Every illness impacts on your physical condition. Your doctor must also know what drugs you are taking, legal or illegal, prescription or non-prescription. Drug interactions can be lethal. You accomplish nothing by concealing this kind of information. Finally, there is no reason to conceal visits to other doctors. Your doctor needs to be told why you consulted other professionals and what they told you. There have been reported cases, recently, of people who have died of drug reactions caused by using prescriptions from several doctors. It is senseless to put yourself into that kind of jeopardy. Participating in the recordkeeping will also help you to both expand your medical vocabulary and understand how your body works. This, in turn, will improve your ability to ask good questions and understand good advice.

The form (p. 148) was designed so that you could bring together all your medical records in one convenient history. Take the time to fill it out completely. If you do not now have a personal doctor, retain the records until you select one and then give him a copy. If you have a personal doctor, fill out the form carefully and ask him to keep a copy in his records. The form requires considerable effort on your part. The time you spend updating your history could save your life.

Collaborating in the Search for Information

The first step. Most of the contact you will have with your doctor will be in the office or clinic. Use your preparation form to guide your opening statements and refer to it as you are asked questions. Assign priorities. Tell your doctor about the most bothersome problems first. Do not expect him to detect problems he cannot see or you don't talk about.

Do not conceal information. The advantage in having a doctor, as opposed to a veterinarian, is that doctors *do* respond to communication. Even if you feel intimidated, you cannot permit apprehension to prevent you from asking questions or providing personal information. Doctors talk all day, every day, about intimate body parts and private functions. They have "heard it all."

The examination. The second step may involve an examination, although many conditions can be diagnosed without it. There are a number of procedures your doctor can conduct in his office. In addition to a physical exam, most doctors check pulse and blood pressure, do simple urinalysis and blood sugar tests. Some doctors have the facilities to perform electrocardiograms and rectum and colon examinations.

As the doctor proceeds with the examination, you are expected

YOUR PERSONAL MEDICAL HISTORY

Vital Statistics

Date this form was filled out _____

Your name _____

Residence address _____ Phone _____

Business address _____ Phone _____

Who should be notified in the event of emergency? (List two or three)

_____

_____

Date of birth _____ Place of birth _____

Anything special about your birth? (Caesarian, mother had problem pregnancy, used DES, etc.) _____

_____

Marital status _____

Children (List names, birth dates, are they living at home)

Personal Profile

What exactly do you do on your job? _____

(List all the jobs you have held and describe what you did. The kind of work you did and the conditions in which you did can often provide important clues to diseases you may acquire later in life. Use as much space as you need in this section.)

_____

Hobbies _____

What do you enjoy doing most? _____

Do you use alcohol? _____ If "yes," how much, how often, in what form? _____

Do you smoke now? _____ What do you smoke? _____

How much per day? _____

Did you ever smoke? _____ From when to when? _____

Why did you stop? _____

Do you use any recreational drugs? _____ Specify _____

Do you use alcohol? _____ How much and how often?

_____

Your Family Medical History

Father _____ Age _____

Present medical condition _____

Date of death _____ Age at death _____

Cause of death _____

What medical conditions did he have? _____

What surgery did he have? _____

Mother _____ Age _____

Present medical condition _____

Date of death _____ Age at death _____

What did she die of? _____

What medical conditions did she have? _____

What surgery did she have? _____
What can you recall about the health of your grandparents?

_____
_____
_____

Aunts and Uncles? _____
_____
_____
_____

Your Medical History

Your present doctors' name and location _____

REPORT ON EACH DOCTOR YOU HAVE SEEN OR ARE SEEING. Try to
recall as many as you possibly can. Make copies of this form if you
need more.
1. Doctor's name _____
    Approximate date of visit _____
    What did you see him/her for? _____
    Do you have your records from these visits? _____
    What was the outcome? _____
    Why did you stop seeing this doctor? _____
2. Doctor's name _____
    Approximate date of visit _____
    What did you see him/her for? _____
    Do you have your records from these visits? _____
    What was the outcome? _____
    Why did you stop seeing this doctor? _____
3. Doctor's name _____
    Approximate date of visit _____
    What did you see him/her for? _____
    Do you have your records from these visits? _____
    What was the outcome? _____
    Why did you stop seeing this doctor? _____
4. Doctor's name _____
    Approximate date of visit _____
    What did you see him/her for? _____
    Do you have your records from these visits? _____
    What was the outcome? _____
    Why did you stop seeing this doctor? _____
5. Doctor's name _____
    Approximate date of visit
    What did you see him/her for? _____
    Do you have your records from these visits? _____
    What was the outcome? _____
    Why did you stop seeing this doctor? _____
List your childhood diseases

Disease   At what age did it occur?

_____   _____
_____   _____

_____   _____
_____   _____

List chronic conditions you now have

Disease   Date diagnosed: What are you doing for it?
_____   _____
_____   _____
_____   _____

Accidents and injuries

Nature of injury   Date and circumstances
_____   _____
_____   _____
_____   _____

Surgery

Nature of   Date and circumstances
operation
_____   _____
_____   _____
_____   _____

DESCRIBE YOUR CURRENT PROBLEM

Describe the symptoms
  What happens? _____
  _____
  How often? _____
  Under what circumstances? _____
  _____

Has it ever happened before? _____ Circumstances _____
_____

Have you ever spoken to a doctor about it? _____
  When? _____
  Circumstances _____
  _____

What physical, laboratory, or X-ray findings were there? _____
_____

What did your doctor say was the problem? What was its cause?
_____

What were you told to do: What did you do: What happened?
_____

Does it affect what you normally do? _____
In what way? _____

to follow instructions, although it is reasonable to ask the doctor what she is doing and what she is looking for. Since most doctors see their mission as instructional, they will be happy to fill you in. In fact, they learned by watching and listening to their supervisors explain what they were doing while examining patients. The doctor's explanation may prompt you to provide information you may have overlooked during the history.

Tests. Your doctor may not be able to make a diagnosis right away. Tests may be required. Be sure you understand the nature and purpose of the tests. Ask about costs, where the tests will be taken, when the reports will be back, and how you can get the information. Try to recall similar tests you have taken. Mention it to your doctor if you have had dental Xrays recently, if he suggests you need X rays now.

Laboratory tests are expensive. Controversy surrounds random testing. Some doctors, apprehensive about possible malpractice suits, require more tests than they need to make a diagnosis. Others require tests because they are cautious. You have the right to answers to the following questions: Why must I take the test? What are you looking for? How will it contribute to the diagnosis? Is it dangerous? What will it cost? Will insurance cover it? Are there other ways to get the same information? If so, why don't you use them? How reliable is the test? How reliable is the laboratory?

Some tests are trivial and cause minimum discomfort and inconvenience. Other tests are as risky as minor surgery. Be sure you know where to go for the test and how long it will take. Some tests require special preparation, for example, tests for diabetes or intestinal X rays. If your test requires a special appointment, make sure your doctor makes it for you.

Waiting for test results can be suspenseful and annoying. Tests given late in the week may require you to wait over a weekend for results. Arrange in advance how and when to get the test results. Test results can be given over the phone, though sometimes the length of explanation requires an appointment. Be sure you have this follow-up arranged before you go for the tests. If either you or your doctor is going to be delayed or out of town when the results come in, arrange a way to get the results.

Diagnosis. A diagnosis is usually possible after the history, examination, and testing. Your doctor should either be able to reassure you that nothing is wrong, that there is no change in an existing condition, or be able to identify what you have and explain how he knows you have it. Inquire about how you might have acquired the disease, what its natural course is, and where you are in the cycle. While your doctor cannot predict the future, he should have general information about the disorder and be able to offer you a best-case, worst-case, and most-likely-case scenario of the illness.

If you want more information about your condition, consult your public library. Your doctor may have pamphlets on the subject or you may be able to get information from an organization that provides information on that condition. If you don't understand what you read, ask your doctor to clarify matters, even if this requires another appointment.

Advice. Advice follows diagnosis. This can include doing nothing, taking medication, altering your life-style, more tests, a visit to a specialist, hospitalization, or surgery. You need not accept a single recommendation. No matter what your doctor recommends, ask about alternatives. Except for serious emergencies, there are usually alternatives in treatment and you should be the one to choose.

If your doctor recommends you do nothing, ask about the ordinary course of the problem. Find out what you can expect and make arrangements to report if anything unexpected happens. If you have a common cold, going home and resting in bed may be all that is necessary. On the other hand, if the symptoms get worse or the cold hangs on longer than usual, you will need to contact your doctor.

Medications. Medications are the most common form of treatment. Almost everyone expects to come out of the doctor's office with a prescription in hand. We pointed out in chapter 4 that a number of doctors have patients for whom they prescribe medication because they know the patient would be dissatisfied without it, not because it is warranted.

It is not wise to pressure your doctor for a prescription. If medication is prescribed, know all you can about it. Your pharmacist can provide some information, but you must be sure of the crucial information before you leave the doctor's office. Find out the name of the medication. Get its trade name and its generic name. Ask if a generic is all right (they are usually less expensive), and if not, find out why the brand name drug is superior. Find out if it is a tranquilizer, an antibiotic, sedative, laxative, etc. Learn what the medication does to your body and what it is supposed to do about your problem. Inquire how long it takes the substance to do its work, and when you should report if you are not feeling better in a reasonable time.

Some prescriptions palliate, others cure. If you have a bacterial infection, the antibiotic may work on the cause but it may not make you feel better quickly. You may still have to take aspirin and force fluids. Your doctor should make all this clear.

Make sure your doctor checks the instructions and you check them again with the pharmacist. If the instructions your pharmacist puts on the bottle conflict with those given by your doctor, do not take the medication: call the doctor. Make sure you know how many pills, tablets, or spoonfuls you take, how often, at what time of day, and under what circumstances. Some prescription drugs must be taken with food, others cannot. Specific foods may alter the effectiveness of some drugs. Still, others may interact with drugs you are currently taking. Check all this before you leave the doctor's office and check it again with your pharmacist.

Despite the fact that most doctors and pharmacists are careful about medications, errors can occur. Most medications are reliable if taken properly. However, all medications have possible side effects. The Food and Drug Administration (FDA) requires that medications be carefully tested on animals and clinically tested in double blind studies on humans before they are authorized for sale. The animals are used to check toxicity and tolerance limits. The double blind tests compare the results in patients, half of whom are getting a placebo (sugar pill) while the other half get the drug that is being tested. No one knows which is which, even the participating doctors. When the testing is over, doctors have a pretty good idea of the drug's effectiveness, its contraindications (when it should not be used), and its side effects. Doctors then file reports on the effects of medication on their patients, and updates of drug information are regularly issued. Make sure your physician keeps up to date and urge him to provide you with the most current information on the drugs you use.

Some doctors are reluctant to supply information about side effects. They worry that knowing the possible side effects will suggest symptoms. Exercise your option to know. Sometimes the side effects are more severe than the condition the drug is supposed to alleviate.

On occasion, as with chemotherapy treatment for cancer, the disease itself is serious enough to demand heroic treatment. The chemicals used to treat cancer are highly toxic. They are, in essence, poisons and have unpleasant effects on the body. When the doctor prescribes them, he must estimate the odds that the poisons will kill the bad cells before they wipe out the good cells. The situation is just that tight. Patients who take the drugs often experience severe discomfort.

Changes in life-style. Your doctor may recommend major changes in your life style in addition to, or instead of, medication. If so, be sure you understand what you are supposed to do, why the doctor believes it will improve your condition, and how long it will be before you see some results. Major life-style changes are tough to make. Yet, diabetics, people with cardiac conditions, and arthritics, to name a few, must do so, if they are to experience a reasonable quality of life. Some of the more frequent recommendations include changing eating patterns, exercise, altered work patterns, physical therapy, and psychotherapy.

Changing eating habits is extraordinarily hard, yet crucial in the treatment of many diseases. Inactive people find it very hard to sustain exercise programs. Physical therapy and psychotherapy require considerable emotional and financial commitment. Support groups offer another approach. If you have to give up smoking, for example, or embark on a different eating plan, sharing your plight with others in the same boat can be useful. Ask your doctor where you can find such groups and how to use them.

Specialists. Your personal doctor will usually be a general practitioner of one sort or another. Those who practice family medicine, internal medicine, general practice, and pediatrics are generalists. Sometimes, when they reach the limit of their knowledge and experience, they may need to call in another doctor for a consultation. Chapter 2 acquainted you with the various kinds of specialists. When it is necessary for you to see one, use your personal physician as both ombudsman and interpreter. Even if you have to see a specialist regularly, it is important to maintain the connection with your personal physician, who, of course, will be alert to the possibility of other conditions developing.

Your personal physician should contact the consulting specialist. He will share important information about your case with the specialist and arrange to have reports transmitted. While the specialist will usually inform you about your condition carefully and in detail, your personal physician can integrate the specialized information into your whole history and discuss implications and possibilities.

Surgery. If your doctor recommends surgery, you should be especially alert. Surgery is never trivial. If the recommendation is made, you must ask a series of questions.

—What is the reason for the surgery? What condition will be modified? Why is this modification necessary?

—Are there alternatives? What will happen if the surgery is not performed? Are there medical procedures that might be effective?

—What exactly will happen during the surgery?

—What are the risks? What are the odds that the surgery will be effective? What possible complications are there?

—Who is available to do the surgery? What place provides the best surgeons? (You have alternatives. Ask for them.)

—Is it a hospital procedure or can it be done on an outpatient basis?

—Roughly how long will I be laid up? How long is the recuperation time at home?

—How long will I be followed after the surgery?

When you have satisfactory answers to all these questions, seek a second opinion and use it as a basis of comparison. Most doctors encourage second opinions. Some will refer you to another physician in whose expertise they feel confident. You may want to select your own doctor for a second opinion. In any case, be sure your doctor is willing to share basic information about you with the doctor giving the second opinion. Second opinions are sometimes costly and they require a delay in time, but they are essential in all but the most urgent conditions. You should understand fully the consequences of not having the surgery. If you are prepared to live with the condition the surgery is supposed to remedy, you have the right to refuse surgical treatment. On the other hand, if there is no alternative, be sure you have the very best surgeons available.

Hospitalization. Sometimes hospitalization is required to perform tests that cannot be done on an outpatient basis. Your doctor may want to keep you in controlled conditions to try out a treatment or observe your reactions carefully. Newly diagnosed diabetics are often hospitalized so the doctor can work out the proper dosage of insulin. Heart patients are often hospitalized briefly to monitor heart function.

Most often, hospitalization is required when your condition is so serious it cannot be adequately treated at home. Occasionally, hospitalization will be done for an emergency. If you are alert at the time you are sent to the hospital, you should know the reason, the name of the hospital to which you are being sent, and something about its reputation. This is particularly important in large cities, where there are several hospitals. In smaller communities where there is little or no choice, you will still want to know that the hospital is properly accredited and that necessary services are provided. On occasion, it may be more sensible to be hospitalized far away from home, particularly if you need specialized services available at only a few places. Insist that your doctor give you enough information to make an informed choice.

Once you agree to hospitalization, acquaint yourself with the admitting procedure. When do you go in? What should you take with you? What kinds of treatment will you receive? What tests will be performed? How will your doctor keep in touch with you? What is his schedule of rounds? Who else will be dealing with you? What role will be played by nurses, dietitians, therapists, laboratory personnel, and others? What is the visiting schedule?

If you have never been hospitalized, your first contact can be very bewildering. It may seem that hospitalization requires you to give up all your rights. This is not so. You must consent to hospitalization and you must consent to treatment. If you are not satisfied with the treatment you are receiving, you have the right to be cared for elsewhere. You also have the right to complete information. In many hospitals, nurses and ancillary personnel are carefully trained to provide information. However, if you are not getting adequate information, your personal physician should be able to provide it for you, and make it easier for you to get it from hospital personnel.

What happens to you in the hospital is carefully controlled. You will be asked to eat the hospital diet, to submit to tests and measurements, and to follow hospital protocol. Much of this regimentation is necessary to efficient operation of the hospital, but it may also be required by the gravity of your condition. You would not be in the hospital if your condition was not serious enough to warrant it. Your informed consent to hospitalization implies informed consent to the course of treatment your doctor specifies. All hospital personnel will follow your doctor's orders and they will not modify them without his approval. That is another important argument for having a personal doctor in whom you have confidence.

Make good use of the time your doctor spends with you in the hospital. If possible, keep written notes and discuss your questions and requests daily during his visits. It is not helpful to get involved in arguments or disagreements with hospital personnel. They have very few alternatives about what they do, and they can make your stay much more comfortable if you cooperate with them and understand the limitations on what they can do.

Follow-up. Follow-up is a crucial part of the relationship with your personal physician. Regardless of the outcome of any particular visit, follow-up is usually necessary. Most doctors have standard routines for providing you with information and for answering your questions. Inquire about how it is most effectively done. Most follow-up can be done by phone. When you have been given a prescription, it is important to check back and let the doctor know how the treatment is going. Find out at the time you receive the prescription when you should call and what you should report. Be sure you know how to report side effects.

After hospitalization, expect one or more follow-up office visits to check on your progress. Your doctor will tell you when to get an appointment. It is convenient to make the appointment before you leave the office, so that both of you can schedule your time efficiently.

Emergencies. It is especially important to know how your doctor handles a change in your condition or an emergency. Find out whether your doctor will talk with you or whether information is to be routed through the nurse or receptionist. Be sure you know what to do if after-hours calls are necessary, or if you need to call when the doctor is off. Most doctors arrange to have their calls covered. If your doctor does not have such arrangements, find another doctor. Illnesses do not respect the schedules of either doctors or patients. Therefore, avoid doctors who do not have routines for handling phone calls and emergencies and who do not arrange coverage, when they are not available. Next to communication, the most important aspect of medical care is availability.

Financial Considerations

In the previous chapter we pointed out that financial considerations represented a major barrier to a productive medical relationship. Patients would prefer not to think about themselves as economic units. But if doctors do not act with fiscal prudence, they do not survive economically. There are a few doctors who accept salaried positions or go into research, but the bulk of American medicine is practiced by independent entrepreneurs, each of whom operates his practice privately. Doctors set their own fees, decide on what equipment to buy, set their own rules of practice, and impose their own criteria for the selection of patients.

Cost considerations should not deter you from seeking the care you need. Most doctors charge reasonably for their time. They must see a minimum number of patients to meet overhead. The most recent calculation for internists, family practitioners, and pediatricians is 115 to 120 patients per week, which, at current fees, figures to about $140,000 a year with four weeks off for vacation and continuing education. Hospital visits might add another $30,000 to $40,000. Rent and utilities for the typical office in an ordinary suburb would come to about $27,000 a year, malpractice insurance would run roughly $10,000 (a low estimate for internists and general practitioners only; others would be considerably higher). A receptionist and a nurse require salary and benefits totaling about $40,000 a year. Subtract regular costs for supplies, bookkeeping, medical journals, equipment maintenance, maintenance on the office, and whatever else it costs to run a business plus purchase of medical insurance and retirement annuities (since physicians do not get employee benefits), and you find the typical physician nets somewhere in the vicinity of $90,000 a year, before income tax. Some specialists, of course, earn considerably more, but all things considered, fees for service charged by the typical physician do not appear quite so high. Consider the prices in a current (1987) physician supplies catalogue:

Economy model (electrocardiograph, table top model)	$1,279.00
Deluxe tabletop model	$3,168.00
Disposable exam gloves	$9.00/100
(The typical doctor uses about 300 gloves per month.)	
Ultrasonic cleaner (for stainless steel equipment)	$ 266.00
Office scale	$ 251.35
Binocular microscope	$ 929.50
Examining table	$1,615.00
Diagnostic fiber-optic pocket set	$ 205.64
Fiber-optic sigmoidoscope	$2,344.95
Digital thermometer	$ 364.46
Sterilizer	$1,655.21
Stethoscope	$ 134.90
Mercury blood pressure kit (sphygmomanometer)	$ 159.00

There is no way to escape financial considerations in securing medical care. On the other hand, you must not be deterred from seeking the medical care you need because of your fear of the cost.

Most doctors serve some nonpaying patients and are willing to make arrangements for their own patients who are temporarily unable to pay.

LETTER TO MRS. H. (A NINETY-YEAR-OLD PATIENT)

Dear Mrs. H.:

My secretary told me that you called three times this week about your bill. I have already informed you that I do not accept Medicare assignment and I expect my patients to pay me and fill out their own insurance forms. Nevertheless, my secretary is always ready to help you do this. She has helped you with seven forms in the first three months of this year. Anytime you are unable to pay, discuss it with me. I will work it out. Please come see me as we discussed during your last visit. You are a valued patient. We all look forward to seeing you 24 April 1987.

Sincerely,
William J., M.D.

Doctors who accept charity patients have the option to fill out complicated forms for minimal payment or give the care free of charge. On the other hand, they are not obligated to take patients who cannot pay unless they are on the staff of a hospital built with Hill-Burton funds. This includes most of the community and teaching hospitals in the country. Physicians on the staff of those hospitals must take charity patients as a condition of membership. The thought that you must pay money for care when you are feeling miserable is somewhat hard to swallow, but it is a fact of life. On the other hand, recent trends in financing medical care through third-party payers have made medical care in some form available to almost everyone.

Learning about Insurance

Third-party payers have revolutionized the financing of medical care. The term refers to any organization involved in financing medical services other than the patient and the doctor. The federal government, for example, pays for military dependents under

CHAMPUS and for the elderly under Medicare/Medicaid. Private companies offer a variety of forms of coverage, the best known of which is Blue Cross/Blue Shield. Financing can also be provided under a Health Maintenance Organization (HMO) or Preferred Provider Organization (PPO). By necessity, imposition of a third party generates paper work for both doctors and patients. Most doctors require their patients to manage their own insurance forms. Some doctors provide a "super bill," a complete statement acceptable to most insurance companies. A few will still fill out forms for patients so they can be paid directly by the insurance companies.

You have a great many insurance options. Your employer may provide health insurance as an employee benefit. Or you may buy health insurance direct from private companies. It is possible to combine coverage by purchasing coinsurance that covers the portion of the medical bill that is not covered by the primary insurance policy.

Some doctors will accept insurance company limits in setting their fees. Others will render an additional bill over and above the coverage. Some policies have a deductible feature, that is, they will only cover the bills after you have paid a specified sum.

If your doctor requires you to file for reimbursement, it is said he or she does not "accept assignment." When your doctor accepts payment directly from the payer, he is said to "accept assignment." The amount paid for services is determined by the doctor before the care is rendered. Regardless of what your insurance company covers, you are responsible for the whole bill. Currently, the main exception to this is the physician who "accepts assignment" from Medicare. In that case, the doctor and Medicare have agreed in advance what the fee and direct reimbursement will be, and the patient has no say or responsibility. You are responsible for understanding your own coverage. There are so many different forms, it would be impossible for your doctor to keep posted on all of them.

When you buy health insurance, buy carefully. There are five major forms of medical insurance currently available in the United States: traditional private insurance, prepaid health plans such as Health Maintenance Organizations (HMO), Preferred Provider

Organizations (PPO), public assistance plans, and government-sponsored insurance for the elderly (Medicare/Medicaid).

Traditional private insurance can be purchased by anyone at any time, if you are eligible. Be careful to check policies for exclusions of preexisting conditions. Be especially careful of insurance policies for specific diseases. Most insurance carriers provide general policies that cover a wide range of services including doctor visits, hospitalization, drugs, therapy, and medical equipment. On the other hand, the more coverage you want, the more costly the policy. Furthermore, most insurance policies will include some kind of deductible feature, that is, they will begin to pay for care only after you have paid a specified sum out of pocket.

To purchase insurance, you simply go to an insurance agent or apply to an insurance company for the plan that you think best meets your needs or fits your budget. When you are covered by a company policy be especially careful to discover what happens at retirement. Most company policies permit retirees to continue their policies at their own expense, but there is usually a time limit within which you must act.

Organizations like the American Association of Retired People and most fraternal and professional organizations offer their members group plans at reduced rates. These insurance plans either pay a portion of the doctor's fee or pay you directly in the event of illness or hospitalizations. They are useful when you have a high deductible, because they will pay regardless of other coverage.

On the other hand, people on Medicare must be very cautious about purchasing supplementary insurance. Most health insurance plans will not cover what Medicate does not cover. It is important to understand policy inclusions—whether payments are direct to provider or cash supplements, and whether particular conditions and treatments are excluded. Recent media campaigns advertising medical insurance to the elderly can generate unnecessary anxieties.

Insurance plans range from limited to comprehensive. Limited plans cost less but usually cover only basic expenses. Read your policy carefully. You should be covered for expensive hospital-related items like the daily cost for a hospital room in your area, diagnostic tests, physician hospital visits, costs of surgery, medications, special nursing services, laboratory tests, operating room costs, medications, anesthesia, emergency room visit costs, X rays, and support services. Be sure you know the prevailing costs in your area before you buy insurance, and make sure your plan is sufficient to meet them. Most plans operate on a deductible basis, and you must take into account how much you can afford to pay at one time and compare it with the cost of your insurance per month or year in order to make a sensible decision. A call to your local hospital is all it takes to discover the exact fees.

Insurance plans can also cover office visits to your doctor, emergency visits to office or clinic, outpatient diagnostic costs, outpatient procedures, psychotherapy and counseling, dental care, optometric (eye) care, podiatric (foot) care, among other things. When selecting your policy go over all the covered costs and evaluate them against your projected needs. Consult a reliable insurance agent if you have questions about coverage. Avoid an insurance agent that will not discuss the details of coverage with you or let you read the policy before you make the first payment.

This same reasoning applies to those who have medical insurance as a benefit of employment. You must realize that no matter what you were told about your policy at employee orientation, the insurance company has to live up to the terms of the policy. You should have access to your policy and you should read it carefully. If it does not appear to cover what you need, there may be nothing you can do about it—your employer buys a group policy and everyone is covered the same way. But you may want to purchase additional insurance to meet your personal needs.

If you have trouble understanding your policy, have your insurance agent interpret it for you. Pay him a fee to explain it to you. It is *your* responsibility to understand your medical insurance. If you are satisfied with what your employer is providing, you need do nothing more except pay attention if the company announces they are changing the coverage. If you find the employer's offering does not cover all you would like, you have the option to buy additional insurance.

Be careful with supplemental policies. Some may not cover you, if you have other insurance. Furthermore, some are inexpensive but may not provide the coverage you want or need. Some bargain policies, for example, might cover "Parkinson's disease." If you buy that policy at the age of twenty-one, you will probably pay at least nineteen years of premiums before you are even in danger of getting the disease, and since the disease is relatively rare, your chances of getting it are slim even then. Furthermore, supplemental policies sometimes do not pay immediately and if you are dependent on them, you may have to make provision for loans to carry you through. Also, some supplemental policies may invalidate portions of the insurance your employer provides. Insurance salesmen are no more likely to try to cheat you than any other merchant, but remember, they are trying to make a sale. It is sensible to figure out your insurance coverage when you are well rather than discover too late that you are not covered.

Prepaid health plans must also be considered carefully. They offer some form of financial coverage of medical care under prearranged rules. These plans may offer more or less than traditional insurance. The ones offering more usually cost more than traditional plans. The bottom line is to know exactly what is being offered, under what terms, and at what cost.

For example, HMOs usually are organized to provide comprehensive medical care for you (and sometimes your family) anytime you need it, but only through a group of practitioners who provide service within the plan. You pay a flat monthly fee to belong to the HMO and no matter what your medical condition, you pay no more. The organization provides the building and people to give you medical care. You will be seen by one or more doctors as needed on each visit. But you are confined to the doctors that participate in the plan. If you need services not provided by the plan you are required to pay for them as provided in the plan.

If you need hospitalization you will be admitted to the hospital owned by or associated with the HMO. Once you are in the hospital, you will see the doctor assigned to your case. If you have complaints about your care you will have to use the administrative procedures provided by the plan. If you choose to go elsewhere for care, nothing is covered. You pay everything outside of the plan out of your own pocket.

A PPO, on the other hand, enlists the services of a number of doctors as "preferred providers." You may choose any one of them to care for you and your expenses are covered anywhere from 80 percent (in most cases, sometimes less) to 100 percent. The doctors in a PPO agree to lower their standard fees in exchange for a guaranteed flow of patients, not a small matter in times of increasing doctor competition.

In addition, if you need hospitalization, you will be admitted to one of the hospitals associated with the PPO. Your expenses will be covered 100 percent. If you choose another hospital, the PPO will pay part of your expenses. If you do not require a long, intensive hospitalization, this drawback is not significant. Your PPO usually covers 60 to 80 percent of the costs in a noncovered hospital (if your bill is $2,000, you will pay $800 of it—a substantial sum but not out of reach for most people). On the other hand, a $23,000 bill could cost you $9,200. There are usually arrangements in case you have emergencies, if you are traveling outside your home region. If you are covered by or contemplate HMO or PPO coverage, it is still important to read the provisions of the plan carefully, just as you would do with an insurance policy.

In the past few years competition for patients has increased. HMOs, PPOs, and medical groups compete with private physicians for the patient dollar. This sometimes results in improved medical care. Even so, the pressure of competition sometimes drives costs up, dehumanizes the contact between doctors and patients, and actually results in less care being available. Before joining a special plan, be sure you know what it covers and what it excludes. Inquire how it works if you should become ill away from home and what access you have to specialized medical facilities. Be especially careful about surrendering your right to free choice of physicians and hospitals.

The federal government provides Medicare to retired persons and Medicaid for the indigent. Most states provide additional plans for both groups. Local communities also provide services, as do a great many private eleemosynary groups. Since a great many people do not receive medical care because they do not understand their coverage, we urge you to check with the proper agency in your area. Both your state Office of Aging and your federal Social Security Office will have information on public programs. Be especially careful to comply with enrollment deadlines and follow procedures for enrollment carefully. In filing claims, take extreme care to do the paperwork correctly. Furthermore, with medical costs rising, it is important to have some coinsurance plan to back up your public coverage.

In summary, no matter what medical plan or insurance you have or are considering, read the fine print. If the language confuses you, hire an expert to interpret it for you. It is essential that you understand your medical plan; it is too late when they are wheeling you into your hospital room. Be sure your personal physician and the staff know your coverage. Be sure you know how your doctor processes third-party payments. Some doctors are willing to fill out the forms and take direct payment from the insurance company. Others expect you to pay, though they will fill out the forms for you. They will give you proof of payment along with a medical report you can send in with your claim. Still others will put the entire burden of making the claim on you. Financial arrangements are an important part of your relationship and you should be completely informed on the procedures.

Understanding Your Doctor

Your doctor is neither hero nor saint. Whatever you have learned to expect from doctors in general, you must understand your own doctor in the context of your relationship. Understand how he works, evaluate how he treats you and how effective the treatment has been. Expect courtesy and consideration but do not count on developing a special relationship.

To your physician, you are part of a day's work. Once Mr. Brown's common cold is diagnosed, and Mrs. Burke is sent off to the hospital to get her appendix out, and Mr. Spencer is shown how to give himself an insulin injection, and a phone call is made to check on Mrs. Wagner in intensive care, there is Mrs. Gottleib's gall bladder and Mr. Cramer's heart and a couple of cases of flu in the waiting room.

And then to the hospital to check a patient in intensive care and look in on a few convalescents: instructions for Mr. Blake to go home, medications arranged for Mr. Hooper, and then home to dinner; the paper, a little TV, and then the phone calls start. Mrs. Clark is still complaining about her cystitis and Mr. Hacker worries a little about his emphysema. Then to bed, only to wake up at 2:00 A.M. to Mrs. Wheeler whose son Freddy is having another of his late-night asthma attacks and up again at 4:00 A.M. to the phone call from the intensive care unit about Mrs. Wagner. And so it goes with your doctor, day after day.

PATRICK Z., M.D. (INTERNIST), AGED FORTY-FOUR

No one except a physician can truly understand the pressures and demands a practice places on us. Not even my parents who have long supported my aspirations seem to understand. The worst thing is not death, dying, keeping up, but the constant availability. You are never really off work unless you are out of town without a phone. It's like the Chinese water torture: one or two drops of water in the face is tolerable, even pleasant, but after two weeks each waterdrop is a hammer blow. Knowing that the phone may ring at any moment and demand you stop what you are doing jangles your nerves so much that you never relax unless there is no phone or beeper. Unless you experience this firsthand, you cannot understand. It's no wonder doctors tend to discuss doctoring at social gatherings with other doctors. With whom else can you commiserate?

You get sick, recover, and get on with your life. Your sickness is a small part of your doctor's routine. To survive, he must put each case in perspective. He cannot give too much emotion to any one individual. There must be enough to go around.

If you wonder why doctors live that way, it is because they love it. They love the intellectual challenge, the physical demands, and the social and economic rewards. They can make it work only by maintaining a reasonable distance from their patients. They must care enough about you to do their best, but not so much that they are distracted from their other patients. On the other hand, some physicians cannot take it. The rate of mental breakdown, drug addiction, family breakup, and suicide among physicians is higher than in the general population. As a patient, you must be alert for signs of impairment in your doctor. If your doctor seems no longer able to give you competent and courteous service, it may be time to make a change. It is irrational to remain loyal to a doctor who is no longer functioning adequately.

Specialists have a very different view of your illness. They are concerned with the details and complications, but they depend on your doctor to interpret results and guide your treatment. An oncologist (cancer specialist), for example, deals with death every day. But he has no time for mourning. He must get on to the next case, the one for which there is still some hope.

Changing Doctors

You have no obligation to remain with a doctor whose work you do not find satisfying. You are paying for services and you are entitled to shop until you find the doctor whose personality and method of practice suit you. On the other hand, you will never find a perfect relationship. Too much shifting around can jeopardize the accuracy of your records and prevent your doctor from getting to know you well.

Doctoring works, most of the time. When doctors get accurate information and have the opportunity to check you carefully, they can usually figure out what is wrong and suggest something to do about it. The problem of jumping from doctor to doctor is that each one will only see fragments of your total behavior. Each will have less of a picture of you to work with. Forgive the cliché, but when you don't know history you are doomed to repeat it. The more your doctor knows about what happened to you when you were sick in the past, the less likely it is that he will expose you to treatment that might put you in jeopardy or cause discomfort.

The medical history form we provided earlier in this chapter is essential to your successful relationship with your doctor. If you haven't filled it out, copy it and do so now. Think through your medical history and complete it in detail. Make a copy for your doctor and keep one for yourself. Provide your spouse and dependents with copies, just in case of emergency. The time you spend updating your history could save your life.

Keeping Posted

Medical practice need not be a carefully guarded secret. Doctors seem to know so much more than their patients because the typical patient rarely knows very much about physiology or keeps informed on trends in medicine. It is useful for you to know the vocabulary relevant to your body and how it works. It is also useful to keep a comprehensive medical guide at home. You can use it as a reference as you prepare yourself for a visit to your doctor. We suggest the *A.M.A. Guide* published by Random House or the *Columbia University Guide* distributed by Consumers Union. Or, ask your doctor what guide he would recommend.

You will, of course, continue to see doctors portrayed on television and in the movies and you will hear about this or that breakthrough on the nightly news. When you see or hear something that appears to have some consequence in your case, call your doctor and ask about it. Very often, he will tell you that the news bulletins are premature or the information does not really fit your case. Every so often, a kind of hysteria sets in about a medical discovery. In the fifties, cancer sufferers scrambled madly to get Krebiozin, advertised as a sure cure for their disease. In the seventies, Laetrile got considerable press as the universal cure for cancer. In the eightiess, people are apprehensive about AIDS. Sick people need to have hope but not false hope. Your doctor can give you facts but not miracles. Asking your doctor good questions is the best way to become an expert user of medical care.

Your doctor can help you resist the blandishments of those who try to sell you nostrums and panaceas and to evaluate the many recommendations in popular magazines and the news media about how you can live a healthy life. Should you take fish oil to have a healthy heart? Will eating fiber foods really prevent colon cancer? How important are regular Pap smears? How can you protect yourself against osteoporosis? Discuss these matters with your doctor. Do not take it for granted that the information you get in the media is complete, or even basically accurate. Some is, and some isn't. Your doctor is an appropriate consultant. When you visit your doctor, make notes and ask your questions. It may spare you from being disillusioned by an expensive fad treatment and may even save your life.

An Overview of the Medical Transaction

The basis of medical treatment. If you understand the basic principles of the practice of medicine, you will be better able to deal with your doctor. Physiological science advances on a premise that generalizations can be made about how the body operates. Each normal organ does what it is supposed to do and looks like it is supposed to look. An abnormal organ could look all right but function badly. There is no such thing as a perfectly normal body. Each of us deviates from the hypothetical norm. Virtually every body function can be viewed as falling within a range of normal wherein you function properly. When a body process falls above or below that range, it is classified abnormal. Conversely, when you discover something unusual about your body, a pain or a malfunction, it is presumed to relate to some abnormality in body function.

DR. LaVERNE W. (INTERNAL MEDICINE), AGED FORTY

Let's look at a relatively simple situation like "strep throat." A patient comes in reporting, "my throat is really sore. It hurts. I have trouble swallowing." I look at the throat, and it is colored according to the pictures in my textbook and the way I was trained to indicate any sore throat. It used to take a good deal of time to do a culture to be sure, but now there is a short test we can do in the office. So I do the test, and it is positive and I diagnose strep. Then I check the records to see if I have treated this patient with any of the antibiotics we can use against strep. I check both for allergies and effectiveness. Then, to be on the safe side, I ask the patient about past experience with drugs. This is very important in a new patient or a patient I haven't seen very often. In addition to records from other doctors I have to depend on the patient's memory.

I write the prescription and I go over the way it is to be taken. Some antibiotics are taken on an empty stomach, some with food, some you can't take with milk products, you have to be very explicit. Even though the pharmacist writes the instructions on the label I can't count on the patient reading them. I used to use these little slips the A.M.A. put out where you write out the instruction, but I kept finding them in the wastebasket in the waiting room. Patients would literally chuck them as they walked out. I try to get the patient to repeat the instructions back to me. I warn the patient to take the pills till they are all gone because the bacteria can adapt if you don't wipe them out completely. This is clear-cut, but when I can't find something causing the sore throat things become more difficult. When a patient reports a sore throat and I see no redness and feel no tenderness in the lymph nodes, I really don't know what it is. I have to try to associate it with something else. Frequently, when the tests are negative, I treat the symptoms only.

When I do prescribe I am always concerned about allergic reactions and side effects. I have to find a way to tell the patient to report back to me without scaring him. I don't want to say what the side effects could be because some patients will get them because they think I expect it. Some patients don't like to call back. I say, "call my secretary in three days and let her know how you are getting along." Mostly, they don't call. My secretary is trained and she knows when to tell me things are not going right. Sometimes it is important for me to know the treatment is working.

When I'm working with a chronic patient, like someone whose diet I am trying to manage, I sometimes have no feedback at all and really no way to get it. Patients with high blood pressure have me completely at their mercy. After giving them a prescription, I must check them periodically, but often I don't hear from them until they develop something else, come in with a bad cold, or run out of medicine. I don't have the time or facilities to check with these people, and so they must take responsibility for their own treatment and get in touch with me regularly.

The preceding statement from a very careful physician is an excellent summary of the process of treatment. She is discussing a very simple case, but it involves a great deal of concentration on evidence and knowledge. As diagnoses become more complicated and conditions more serious, concentration must become more intense. Notice how dependent your doctor is on information you provide. If you do not provide sufficient information when it is needed, you actually jeopardize your own treatment. If you do not talk about your concerns, you cannot blame your doctor for not taking them into account.

Your doctor should serve you not only as diagnostician but as teacher. He must help you to understand his recommendations about personal care, medication, further tests, surgery, or hospitalization in order for you to make intelligent choices. You cannot afford to rely on the doctor to give you all the necessary information. To get effective treatment, you must assume your responsibility to inquire and maintain contact.

KARL Z. (PROFESSOR OF PHILOSOPHY OF SCIENCE), AGED SIXTY-FOUR

The medical model is a marvelous adaption of science and art. Doctors are trained to be scientists, but they know that their work is mostly technological, that is, they work with individual cases and try to apply generalizations so that they work with individual people. Patients should understand how this works. Let's take it step by step.

First, doctors have generalizations about the body. The generalizations are the result of a lot of work by a lot of scientists. They are about how hearts behave or what effect this drug has on this microbe. Doctors read these generalizations in textbooks and journals or learn about them in conversations with their colleagues. Most doctors try very hard to stay up to date on their generalizations.

When doctors look at an individual case they try to fit it into a generalization they are familiar with. The more specific information the doctor has, the easier it is to classify the condition. Sometimes even specific information does not help because there is no group to accommodate it. Doctors try to learn from individual cases. By sharing information about individual cases they help to form generalizations that may guide them in future applications.

Once a doctor fits a condition to a generalization there is a good guess possible about cause and treatment. Conditions with a similar cause usually respond to similar treatment, which of course, has to be tailored to the particular needs of the patient. Then the doctor has to work carefully with the patient to make sure the treatment is doing its job, doesn't bring more problems, and so on. It is very complicated process that requires a lot of cooperation.

Criteria for a Successful Medical Encounter

1. Did your doctor listen as you explained the problem for which you were seeking help?

2. Did your doctor ask you questions that helped clarify or explain the nature of your problem?

3. Did your doctor give you an opportunity to ask questions or add information to make the information exchanged accurate and complete?

4. Did your doctor check your records to get an insight into you as an individual and to understand your particular medical condition and problems?

5. Did your doctor do a selective examination in order to get information needed to make a diagnosis and recommend treatment?

6. Was your doctor able to tell you what was wrong?

7. If your doctor suggested getting additional information, did he schedule tests or make appointments with a specialist for you?

8. Did your doctor make a specific recommendation for treatment?

9. If a prescription, did you understand the directions for taking it, what to expect when you took, and when and what to report to your doctor?

10. If your doctor suggested modifying habits, did you understand what and why?

11. If surgery was recommended, did you understand what was to be done and for what reason? Did your doctor make arrangements for you to get a second opinion?

If you can answer these questions and the answers satisfy you, then this book has accomplished its goal. The "secret" of quality medical care is to match a conscientious doctor with an informed patient. In this book we have described both. Our advice: find one of the former and try to be the latter. Your life will be better for it.

Appendix
References

Appendix
Scales Used in the Study

The following scale was administered to our patient and doctor respondents. Doctors were asked to record two answers: their own attitude toward the question and the attitude they expected their patient to have. Patients were asked to record their opinion in three categories: their own doctor, doctors in general, and specialists. The categories of response were: U = usually, most of the time, O = occasionally, often enough to notice, R = rarely: N = never.

1. Doctors prescribe too many drugs.
2. Doctors let you decide when to turn off life-support equipment.
3. Doctors respond to individual patient needs.
4. Doctors recommend too much surgery.
5. Doctors set fees based on ability to pay.
6. Doctors are smarter than most people.
7. Doctors make you wait too long in the waiting room.
8. Doctors only socialize with other doctors.
9. Doctors treat people, not diseases.
10. Doctors treat diseases, not people.
11. Doctors rely excessively on high-tech equipment.
12. Doctors are entitled to high income because of educational investment.

13. Doctors have a great deal of money.
14. Doctors allow too little time per patient in office visits.
15. Doctors are detached from their patients.
16. Doctors don't listen to you when you try to talk to them.
17. Doctors ask too many questions when they take a history.
18. Doctors fees are based on the cost of equipment and tests.
19. Doctors prescribe too many drugs.
20. Doctors don't let patients talk enough when they take a history.
21. Doctors respect their patients' confidence.
22. Doctors treat but they do not cure.
23. Doctors make you wait too long for an appointment.
24. Doctors charge a lot because insurance companies pay.
25. Doctors don't give good care to charity patients.
26. Doctors don't explain well how to use prescriptions.
27. Doctors don't handle terminal illnesses well.
28. Doctors have unhappy family lives.
29. Doctors have exchanged bedside manner for machinery and lab tests.
30. Doctors are not reliable about returning phone calls.
31. Doctors visits to you in the hospital are too short.
32. Doctors are rude to other hospital personnel.
33. Doctors tend to avoid personal contact with their patients.
34. Doctors can't keep up with technical innovations in medicine.
35. Doctors prescribe unnecessary X rays and lab tests.
36. Doctors split their fees with specialists and laboratories.
37. Doctors charge too much.
38. Doctors don't give patients enough information about their illnesses.
39. Doctors distort information to make their patients feel better.
40. Doctors cover up for each other to avoid malpractice suits.
41. Doctors rely on surgery to cure diseases.
42. Doctors tend to be arrogant toward their patients.
43. Doctors don't comply with Medicare.
44. Doctors commit suicide more than average.
45. Doctors take care of people even if they can't pay.

46. Doctors depend on lab tests to diagnose patients.
47. Doctors rely on drugs to cure diseases.
48. Doctors treat men better than women.
49. Doctors are preoccupied with their financial investments.
50. Doctors rely on equipment to cure diseases.
51. Doctors usually tell patients the truth about their condition.
52. Doctors never remember your name.
53. Doctors tend to be cool toward their patients.
54. Doctors don't like to treat old people.
55. Doctors encourage patients to solicit second opinions.
56. Doctors' records tend to be incomplete.
57. Doctors' major interest is making money.
58. Doctors cover up for each other.
59. Doctors try to explain things so patients can understand.
60. Doctors are well worth what they cost.
61. Doctors are important in the community.
62. Doctors charge more money than I can afford.
63. Doctors act like they are portrayed on television.
64. Doctors act friendly to their patients.
65. Doctors don't care about their patients' families.
66. Doctors are generally well trained for their professions.
67. Doctors don't pay attention when I talk to them.
68. Doctors don't like to treat poor people.
69. Doctors act like they are superior to their patients.
70. Doctors are cynical about life.

In addition, patients were asked to provide age, occupation, gender, income, occupation, medical history, and health insurance. Doctors were asked to provide information about their medical specialty, kind of practice, and whether they were ever involved in a malpractice action.

The Ideal Patient Scale

The Ideal Patient Scale gave the following instructions to doctors.

When we think of an ideal patient we think of the patient who did his or her best to cooperate with medical treatment. It is not necessarily the patient you liked best or least. It is a patient who did the most to cooperate with you. For your guidance in answering this question, on a separate piece of paper THAT YOU WILL NOT RETURN TO US, identify (by name) a best, worst, and average patient, IN TERMS OF COOPERATION WITH YOU. Use a patient you had within the last year whom you saw both in your office and in the hospital. Use these three names to guide you in your answers to the questions below.

A. What was the diagnosis? (best, worst, typical patient)
B. Describe the patients's demographics (sex, age, race, job, etc.).
C. What did they talk with you about when you made hospital visits?
D. How did they treat nurses and other hospital personnel?
E. What did they talk with you about during office visits?
F. How did they respond to your instructions?
G. What personal things did they tell you about themselves?
H. What personal things did you tell them about yourself?
I. What questions did they ask you?
J. How was the patient's family involved?
K. What did the patient expect of you?
L. What was the outcome of the case?

Review your answers, please, and then, below, write the criteria for an ideal patient.

Waiting Room Scale

Following is the scale we administered to patients while waiting in a doctor's office and a similar sample who had visited a doctor within the past week.

Part I. Answer the following questions by writing the letter of your answer on the line beside the item. Here are your choices.

I think about this issue
A = almost always, about 100% of the time.
B = frequently, about 3/4 of the time.
C = occasionally, about half of the time.

D = rarely, about 1/4 of the time.

E = almost never.

If the item does not relate to you, leave it blank (for example, if you have no children and the item refers to children, or if the item is about your job and you are not working).

___ 1. Getting proper pay for the work I do on my job.

___ 2. Taking my medicine as prescribed for me.

___ 3. Doing regular formal exercise.

___ 4. Looking good.

___ 5. Driving carefully.

___ 6. Being loved by my mate.

___ 7. Drinking too much alcohol.

___ 8. Eating a balanced diet.

___ 9. Following instructions given me by my doctor.

___ 10. Making sure my kids do well in school.

___ 11. Having enough money.

___ 12. Fastening my seat belts when I am in the car.

___ 13. Defects in my body I inherited from my ancestors.

___ 14. Avoiding salt in my food.

___ 15. Getting cancer.

___ 16. Keeping my job.

___ 17. Observing my religious beliefs properly.

___ 18. Having sex.

___ 19. Getting heart trouble.

___ 20. Dressing attractively.

___ 21. Keeping my body fit.

___ 22. Avoiding too much fat in my diet.

___ 23. Enjoying myself from time to time.

___ 24. Having problems with my teeth.

___ 25. Having fun.

___ 26. Having good friends.

___ 27. Spending quality time with my kids.

___ 28. Going to the bathroom regularly.

___ 29. The possibility that no one loves me.

___ 30. Not smoking (or giving up smoking).

___ 31. Being right with God.

___ 32. What my medical care will cost me.

___ 33. What my loved ones will do after I die.

___ 34. Getting AIDS.

___ 35. The possibility of a nuclear war.

___ 36. Not having medical care when I need it.

___ 37. The possibility of being involved in a car wreck

___ 38. Cost of a major hospitalization.

___ 39. The possibility of catching a disease.

___ 40. Doing something worth while for other people.

Part II. Look carefully at each of the following pairs. In each case, find the one you worry about the most and write its letter in the space provided. For example, if you have an item that looks like this:

     ___ 99. A. Buy a new car
              B. Remodel the house

If you want to buy a new car more than remodel the house, write "A" in the space provided. If you want to remodel the house more than buy a car, write "B" in the space provided. *Remember, your job is to decide which one you WORRY ABOUT more.*

The following items were then presented in all possible pairs:

1. Understanding my inherited body characteristics.
2. The way I eat, especially avoiding salt, sweets, and fat.
3. Exercising regularly.
4. Avoiding tobacco and limiting alcohol.
5. Driving safely, especially fastening my seat belt.
6. Being happy and keeping an optimistic outlook on life.
7. Having enough money to pay for what I need and want.
8. Following my religion and being right with God.

References

Cassell, Eric J. *Talking with Patients.* Vol. 1, *The Theory of Doctor-Patient Communication.* Cambridge: MIT Press, 1985.

———. *Talking with Patients.* Vol. 2, *Clinical Technique.* Cambridge: MIT Press, 1985.

Katz, Jay. *The Silent World of Doctor and Patient.* New York: Free Press, 1984.

Kline, Susan L., and Janet M. Ceropski. "Decision Making in the Doctor-Patient Relationship: Interactive Dimensions of the Process." In *Emergent Issues in Decision Making*, ed. Gerald M. Phillips and Julia T. Wood. Carbondale and Edwardsville: Southern Illinois University Press, 1984.

Kreps, Gray L., and Barbara C. Thornton. *Health Communication.* New York: Longman, 1984.

Kunz, Jeffrey R. M., ed. *The American Medical Association Family Medical Guide.* New York: Random House, 1984.

Long, James M. *The Essential Guide to Prescription Drugs.* Bridgeport: Consumer Reports Books, 1986.

Pettegrew, Loyd. *Explorations in Provider and Patient Interaction.* Louisville: Humana, Inc., 1982.

Physicians Desk Reference. Oradell, NJ: Medical Economics Co., Inc., 1987.

Rosenfeld, Isadore. *Modern Prevention*. New York: Simon and Shuster, 1986.

Sehnert, Keith. *How to Be Your Own Doctor (Sometimes)*. New York: Putnam Publishing Co., 1985.

Starr, Paul. *The Social Transformation of American Medicine*. New York: Basic Books, 1982.

Tapley, Donald F., ed. *The Columbia University College of Physicians and Surgeons Complete Home Medical Guide*. Bridgeport: Consumer Reports Books, 1986.

Thompson, Theresa L. *Communication for Health Professionals*. New York: Harper and Row, 1986.

West, Candace. *Routine Complications*. Bloomington: Indiana University Press, 1984.

J ALFRED JONES, M.D., has been engaged in the private practice of internal medicine in State College, Pennsylvania for ten years. Born in Gainesville, Florida, he did his undergraduate work at the University of Florida, majoring in chemistry. He received his M.D. degree at the University of Miami School of Medicine and did his postdoctoral work in internal medicine at the University of Vermont.

GERALD M. PHILLIPS, Ph.D., has been professor of speech communication at the Pennsylvania State University for twenty-four years. He received his B.A., M.A., and Ph.D. degrees at Case-Western Reserve University. Professor Phillips is a specialist in disturbed communication and has written 27 books and 105 articles. He is a former editor of *Communication Quarterly*.

DATE DUE

MAY 19 '96			

Demco, Inc. 38-293